# Efficacy of Special Education and Related Services

By

Kenneth A. Kavale, PhD
University of Iowa

Steven R. Forness, EdD
University of California, Los Angeles

Gary N. Siperstein, PhD
*Editor*

# AAMR
American Association on Mental Retardation

Published by
American Association on Mental Retardation
444 North Capitol Street, NW, Suite 846
Washington, DC 20001-1512

The points of view expressed herein are those of the authors and do not necessarily represent the official policy or opinion of the American Association on Mental Retardation. Publication does not imply endorsement by the editor, the Association, or its individual members.

Printed in the United States of America.

**Library of Congress Cataloging-in-Publication Data**
Kavale, Kenneth A., 1946–
        Efficacy of special education and related services/Kenneth A. Kavale, Steven R. Forness.
                        p. cm. — (Monographs of the American Association on Mental Retardation)
                Includes bibliographical references.
                ISBN 0-940898-51-9
                1. Handicapped—Education—United States—Evaluation.
2. Handicapped students—Services for—United States—Evaluation
3. Mentally handicapped children—Education—Aims and Objectives—
United States.  4. Special education—United States—Evaluation.
I. Forness, Steven R.  II. Title.  III. Series.
LC4031.K38            1998
371.9'0973—dc21                              98-22495
                                                            CIP

# TABLE OF CONTENTS

# FIGURES AND TABLES

## Figures

## Tables

# PREFACE

The basic goals and objectives of special education have not changed substantially since its inception. The primary desire has always been to help individuals with special needs, and the methods used span a wide assortment of activities that may include, for example, mobility training for individuals with visual impairment or designing adaptive devices for individuals with physical disabilities. The majority of special education, however, is delivered in school settings, and this is the focus of the present volume. The interventions to be discussed are based on attempts to enhance the academic, cognitive, and social functioning of individuals with special needs who would otherwise fail in a general education context. To achieve these aims, special education has either developed a variety of unique instructional methods, adapted and modified general education techniques for the purposes of special education, or designed adjunct interventions to foster learning ability. Under its intervention umbrella, special education has also incorporated a number of treatments; take, for example, medications, which are not directly under the purview of teachers or administrators. Special education has also emphasized the prevention of problems with early intervention programs targeted for students at the preschool level.

Special education thus casts a wide net; the breadth of special education suggests that it may take a variety of forms beyond academic instruction. Regardless of its form, special education, almost from the beginning, has met with demands to evaluate its effectiveness. Does special education meet its stipulated goals and objectives in an efficient and appropriate manner? The question has sometimes been phrased: Is special education special? Inherent are questions about whether special methods work, whether the desired outcomes are achieved, and whether the intervention efforts can be justified on a cost-benefit basis.

Special education has developed a substantial research base for judging the effectiveness of its methods and techniques. The difficulty, however, has been in drawing unequivocal conclusions about efficacy. No single study has proved conclusive and neither have reviews attempting to pool the findings from many individual studies. We suggest that the reason for the equivocation is found in the review techniques used. What will be reported here are the findings from integrative reviews using methods of quantitative research synthesis. We believe that these methods, which have come to be known as meta-analyses, provide an objective, explicit, and unambiguous means of drawing more steadfast conclusions from a body of literature.

The findings from a number of meta-analyses are reported. First, meta-analytic findings about the efficacy of methods and techniques that have almost come to define special education are provided. In general, these practices are shown to produce modest effects, calling into question their efficacy. A number of issues that may contribute to the limited effectiveness of special education are discussed. Second, meta-analyses investigating the efficacy of general education practices adapted and modified for the purposes of special education are reviewed. In general, these methods have proven far more effective in producing positive outcomes and suggest differences about the nature of special education with respect to implications about its *special* and *education* components.

The realm of effective instruction is explored and its manifestations for special education described. We conclude that special education, based on principles of effective instruction, can be successful but is often undermined by poor implementation and philosophical disputes surrounding the basic substance of special education practice. We conclude that the effectiveness of special education is a consequence of both science and art. No method is effective or not effective by itself but rather is the result of the special education practitioner's interpretation of best practice.

# ACKNOWLEDGMENTS

The influence of our friends and colleagues in shaping the ideas in this volume cannot be underestimated. A special thank you to Tom Scruggs, Margo Mastropieri, John Lloyd, Jim Kauffman, Shari Vaughn, and Doug and Lynn Fuchs. We alone, however, are responsible for any errors of omission or commission.

Our sincere appreciation for the support and guidance provided by Gary Siperstein. From initial conceptualization to final product, he was instrumental in moving this project forward. It has been a pleasure working with Gary, and we hope we will have similar opportunities in the future.

The efforts of Susan Yoder deserve special recognition. We appreciate her labors in producing this volume.

A special thank you to Erma Statler. From interpreting obscure hieroglyphics to amelioration egregious insult to the King's English, she is always cheerful and cooperative. Her skill was integral to bringing this volume to fruition.

As always, in the very best sense, this is a collaborative effort, and we hope it represents our best insights into the efficacy of special education and related services.

# CHAPTER 1

# SPECIAL EDUCATION AND ITS EFFECTIVENESS

After a decade of relative optimism following passage of Public Law 94-142 in 1975 (now Individuals with Disabilities Education Act), special education over the past decade has found itself under attack as ineffective, costly, and perhaps even immoral, not only in the professional literature but also in the popular press as evidenced by pieces in *U.S. News and World Report* (Shapiro, Loeb, Bowermaster, et al., 1993) and *The Wall Street Journal* ("Special ed's special costs," 1993). This is by no means a new phenomenon, since discussion about efficacy can be traced back to the beginnings of special education with Itard's (1806/1962) work with Victor, the "wild boy" of Aveyron. Although special education possesses a relatively long history, a cursory review can lead to cynicism and despair because change in the form of false hopes and easy solutions has been more characteristic than real change (Kauffman, 1981). The result has been a general pessimism about special education to the point where special education is viewed as harmful, not helpful; evil, not good (Hallahan & Kauffman, 1994). The pessimism surrounding special education was reinforced during the mid-1980s with emergence of the regular education initiative (REI) for students with mild disabilities, which rather rapidly transformed into a full-inclusion movement where all students with disabilities are seen as candidates for full-time instruction in general education classrooms (Fuchs & Fuchs, 1994). The REI focused in large measure on the presumed ineffectiveness of special education instruction (e.g., Reynolds, Wang, & Walberg, 1987; Wang, 1987; Will, 1986); full inclusion, in addition, seems not only to seek complete social and instructional integration (e.g., Lipsky & Gartner, 1989; Snell, 1991; Stainback & Stainback, 1992), but, at the extremes, also to suggest dismantling the entire infrastructure of special education (Pearpoint & Forest, 1992). Thus, the effectiveness of differential services and the quality of instruction emanating from special education are viewed as suspect.

Such lack of effectiveness has been perceived in the context of recent historic changes in special education and disability services (Polloway, Smith, Patton, & Smith, 1996). In this view, transformation from facility-based or special-class services to a more service-based paradigm that prepared persons with disabilities to enter society occurred during the 1960s. Such questioning of the "where" of special education laid the foundation in the 1990s for a supports-based paradigm implicitly critical of special education itself. Such a paradigm is indeed at the heart of the new definition of mental retardation, which focuses not on type or level of disability but on supports needed to ameliorate its effects (Luckasson et al., 1992).

Criticisms about the effectiveness of special education are not always based on empirical evidence. Kauffman and Pullen (1996) have demonstrated how certain myths about disability and special education are accepted uncritically by the special education reform movement. These myths include beliefs that the general education classroom is the most effective learning environment, rewarding students' desirable behavior undermines their intrinsic motivation, effective instruction is effective for all students regardless of their disabilities, and all students benefit from having appropriate social models in the classroom. These myths have been seriously challenged, if not dismissed, and a wide variety of both logical and empirical arguments have been mounted against these and other contentions about special education reform (e.g., Cameron & Pierce, 1994; Hallahan, Keller, McKinney, Lloyd, & Bryan,1988; Hallenback & Kauffman, 1995; Kauffman & Hallahan, 1995; Kauffman & Lloyd, 1995; MacMillan, Gresham, & Forness, 1996; Semmel, Gerber, & MacMillan, 1994).

Although concerns have been expressed about both rising costs and poor outcomes for special education (e.g., Wagner, 1995), recent data suggest that the picture is far less bleak than previously supposed. Analysis of several national cost studies published during the past two decades indicated that total proportionate cost for those receiving special education has changed little (Chaikind, Danielson, & Brauen, 1993). There continues to be concern about transition of adolescents with mental retardation (MR), for example, into work and independent living (e.g., Patton, Polloway, Smith, Edgar, Clark, & Lee, 1996; Smith & Puccini, 1995). Recent findings, however, from a national longitudinal transition study suggested that, although youth with MR lag behind nondisabled counterparts, their rate of competitive employment and independent living has increased significantly in recent years, particularly in the period from 3 to 5 years after schooling (Blackorby & Wagner, 1996).

There is reason to assume, with respect to MR in particular, that such gains coming with little or no increase in costs are especially significant for assessing the effectiveness of special education. It is evident that the rate of identification for MR in schools has continued to decline rather significantly during this same time period (Forness, 1990; Oswald, 1995). This decline is assumed to involve lower identification of students with mild MR, thus leaving primarily those with more severe and multiple disorders populating the MR category. The paradox of improvement on outcome measures during a period when more severe problems are being identified indeed seems significant.

At the same time, there is a certain pessimism about raising the achievement levels of students with MR or related learning problems (Blagg, 1991; Spitz, 1986). The assumption that a substantial amount of MR can be prevented through educational or medical interventions has also been challenged (Stevenson, Massey, Schroer, McDermott, & Richter, 1996). Such apprehension seems by no means reflected in the assumptions behind the current American Association on Mental Retardation (AAMR) definition of MR, where disability appears to mean less a limit on intellectual or functional growth than primarily a need for social and environmental supports to attain such growth (Schalock et al., 1994). This definitional assumption flies in the face of evidence that substantial biologic and comorbid conditions have increased the complexity of challenges for those remaining in the MR category (e.g., Baumeister, Kupstas, & Klindworth, 1990; Bregman, 1991; Bregman & Hodapp, 1991; Forness & Kavale, 1996a). It also flies in the face of concerns that the definition seems very likely to increase the number of students eligible for the MR category, thus potentially burdening special education with additional students in an era of declining resources (MacMillan, Gresham, & Siperstein, 1993, 1995; Smith, 1994).

All of this contention provides a reason to examine once again the research base in special education and its related services to determine whether its procedures, techniques, and methods significantly increase the functioning of students who receive these interventions (Fuchs & Fuchs, 1995a, 1995b). In doing so, it is not always possible to separate out differential effects on children and adolescents with MR, though these results may be of paramount interest to readers. It is clear that, both in special education research and in actual practice, students with disabilities have often been grouped together such that differential outcomes for students with MR, learning disabilities (LD), emotional/behavioral disorders (E/BD), and other disabilities cannot always be determined (Forness & Kavale, 1994; Hewett & Forness, 1984; MacMillan, Siperstein, & Gresham, 1996). The question remains, however, whether special education students attain outcome levels that warrant the continuation of programs and services under the rubric of special education. Depending on individual perceptions, answers may range from a call for the status quo because of perceived benefits derived from special education to a call for radical reform through a restructuring that essentially merges general and special education into a single system serving all students.

# The Meaning of Special Education

For a domain that has generated so much debate, special education is not well-defined. According to federal regulations, special education means "specifically designed instruction, at no cost to the parent, to meet the unique needs of a child with a disability including instruction conducted in the classroom, in the home, in hospitals and institutions, and in other settings; and instruction in physical education" (U.S. Department of Education, 1992). The key words in the definition are *specifically* and *unique:* they represent the basic concept of individualization. The essence of special education

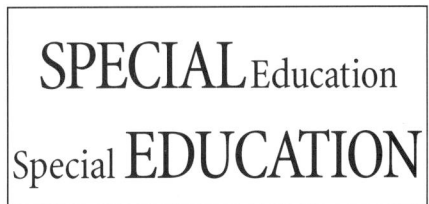

SPECIAL Education

Special EDUCATION

Figure 1. The meaning of special education.

appears to be defined by instruction matched to the particular needs manifested by the individual student. Although individualization is a fundamental concept, the definition does not address the nature of the instruction to be provided. How should individualization be achieved? The ways in which this question is answered, represented in Figure 1, provide insight into the philosophical foundations of special education.

The first response emphasizes the *special* in special education through the development of methods that are unique and exclusive. The techniques developed are not used routinely in general education but are associated with special education only. The second response emphasizes the *education* in special education. Rather than developing methods within the context of special education, existing general education techniques are modified for the purposes of special education. An alternative response would be for general education methods to be used intact but fitted to the individual needs of a special education student. In both cases, the emphasis is on *education* and the use of existing procedures to achieve desired outcomes without relying on techniques that would typically be found only in special education settings.

Given the different emphases, problems in defining special education can be readily discerned. For example, if the *education* part of special education is stressed, is it proper to term these transactions special education, or are they better viewed as an optimal form of general education? To provide a distinct identity and clearly differentiate itself from general education, special education has long opted for an emphasis on the *special*. At one time, special education was essentially defined by the special methods and techniques it developed. Although successful in creating a distinctiveness for special education, the special procedures also introduced a level of separateness that presented only a complementary relationship with general education. The separateness has meant that special education has repeatedly been called upon to prove itself, essentially because it is more labor-intensive and thus expensive, and because general educators have often been skeptical about special education programming (Balow & Brinkerhoff, 1983).

The difficulty created by a separateness between special and general education is found in the fact that, for a majority of special education students, programming is based primarily on the goals and objectives of general education; special education students are required to read, write, spell, calculate, solve problems, and engage in all basic curricular activities. When dealing with populations that possess essentially intact learning processes, special education can closely parallel general education. For example, students with sensory impairments possess learning abilities that are similar to students in general education if the effects of the particular disability (i.e., hearing or visual loss) are accommodated (e.g., sound amplification or enlarged print). Because learning processes are not altered, the enhanced stimulus input permits learning processes to operate efficiently. Special education, under these circumstances, becomes basically a process of accommodation.

The situation becomes more complicated when the special education population does not possess intact learning processes. For the majority of special education students with high-incidence mild disabilities (e.g., MR, LD, E/BD), learning problems in the form of altered learning processes represent the fundamental disability; a common feature of these conditions is school failure caused by a variety of learning disorders. The altered learning functions may result from difficulties with different types of learning (Scruggs, 1988), inactive learning (Torgesen, 1982), or cognitive-motivational problems (Licht, 1983), as examples. Regardless of the cause, the result is the same: a student who does not learn in the ways expected. Under these circumstances, accommodation would not be sufficient. Accommodations must be carefully crafted and individually designed, but their effectiveness is readily judged by whether or not they enable the student to learn in the same way as other students. When, however, learning processes are not intact, accommodation becomes insufficient and must be replaced by a concept like remediation; remediation refers to procedures that correct or reverse something that has gone wrong. Remediation places special education within the context of a medical model, treatment directed at correcting, reversing, or curing what is wrong. Such a framework suggests that learning problems require treatment rather than simply teaching if they are to be over-come.

A concept like remediation, however, with its emphasis on cure, can be in conflict with the goals and objectives of general education instruction. Such differences are what have historically defined special education. If a student requires remediation, then special education, with its remedial methods and techniques, is best equipped to deal with students whose primary difficulties are found in a variety of learning disorders. In theory, the necessity for special education to be *special* through its remedial procedures makes sense, but the effectiveness of these procedures needs to be assessed. Has special education demonstrated sufficient efficacy in its unique procedures to warrant their continuation?

# Research in Special Education

Special education has a long history of empirical research, and large quantities of data have been accumulated. Yet, it has been argued that what passes for the scientific study of human behavior (e.g., special education) is little more than a form of sorcery (Andreski, 1972). Instead of natural and predictable laws to explain phenomena, sorcery posits a sympathetic magic, a primitive view of cause and effect where events are assumed to influence other events even though separated by space, time, and distance. One subset of sympathetic magic, homeopathic magic, is based on the principle of similarity ("like produces like"). When such magical principles are applied to the wrong events in the wrong places, they possess the fatal flaw of unreliability (the magic neither produces nor influences the phenom-enon). Unfortunately, some conceptions in special education have evidenced such magical thinking. For example, the assertion that Doman-Delacato neuro-logical patterning exercises enhance central nervous system organization (see Delacato, 1959) and, consequently, improve language and reading ability represents a form of homeopathic magic.

Research in special education has closely adhered to the "scientific method," which has its roots in logical positivism. The primary assumption of logical positivism is that all knowledge can be accounted for from an empirical and logical perspective without resort to metaphysics; what counts as evidence is "rock-bottom" sense experience (i.e., positive knowledge) (Achinstein & Barker, 1969). The hypothetico-deductive model of logical positivism ("scientific method") has carried the weight of authority, and it has been assumed that only by adhering to its specified sequence can credible findings be obtained. Special education research, like most educational research, has had its credibility judged by the strength of its adherence to the scientific method. Especially for a field viewed as "soft," faithfulness to the scientific method is viewed as necessary if useful knowledge is to be attained (Kavale & Forness, 1994).

Although logical positivism may no longer be a predominant philosophical view (see Eisner, 1983; Phillips, 1983), its influence on the research process remains in the form of "disciplined inquiry" that is distinguished from alternative forms of opinion and belief (Cronbach & Suppes, 1969). In adhering to the scientific method, research in special education produces a numbing sameness, and contributions are judged, not by their content, but rather by the extent to which they parallel the scientific method (Smart & Elton, 1981). Consequently, a rigid and narrow research system is produced that is based on a single, sacrosanct, officially approved methodology. For example, Campbell and Stanley's (1966) classic treatise describes *the* way to do research in special education, and competence is defined only in terms of that research methodology.

The primary difficulty with the scientific method is its emphasis on data collection and analysis over understanding what those data mean. The scientific method creates an "empiricism" that includes large quantities of data that are not joined in any theoretical configuration and thus remain isolated and independent elements without rational connection. The resulting system does not aim at building knowledge cumulatively through a progressive research program but rather seeks the single "perfect" study that will produce universal truth and unassailable facts about, for example, the effectiveness of special education (see Lindblom & Cohen, 1979). No single study can hope to approach this desired

level of perfectness. Each is probably assailable on any number of criticisms that represent the common pitfalls in behavioral research (see Barber, 1976) or the number of "judgment calls" necessary to conduct research even when it is based on the presumed hard and fast rules of the scientific method (see McGrath, Martin, & Kulka, 1982).

Besides careful collection of data, the scientific method also emphasizes data analysis, but there appears to be an overreliance on statistical probabilities in deciding to accept or to reject hypotheses (Carver, 1978). Statistical inference is useful for eliminating chance findings but not nearly as helpful in deciding substantive issues. Techniques of statistical analysis were designed for making practical decisions in applied work that should not be confused with reaching reliable conclusions (Fisher, 1956). Regardless of the sophistication of the statistical analysis, probabilities neither confirm nor refute research hypotheses but only null hypotheses; findings may be "significant," but that significance should not be confused with importance (e.g., Morrison & Henkel, 1970). The difficulty, however, is that caution regarding substantive conclusions is quickly abandoned when probabilities are less than .05. The reverse, however, is not true, and studies with probabilities greater than .05 are neither often published nor given serious consideration (Skipper, Guenther, & Nass, 1967).

The consequences are significant; for example, consider the case where a new special education intervention is compared with an established treatment. Suppose that the new intervention demonstrates a higher mean performance level for the experimental group when compared to the control group, but the obtained mean comparison, with a probability level of .07, is not significant. The new intervention is probably considered a failure (i.e., nonsignificant) and probably does not find its way into the professional literature. Special education, however, has lost valuable information because evidence that might aid decision making is not available. Now suppose that another study (even if methodologically flawed) finds an established treatment more effective than a new intervention, and the mean comparisons are significant with a probability level of .001; in all likelihood, the study is then published in the professional literature. Although it might be only a random finding, the publication of this study makes it the standard and also makes it difficult to eliminate its influence. The new intervention, in the meantime, is relegated to the background and is considered "experimental" without the benefit of a fair and objective evaluation.

# Quantitative Research Synthesis in Special Education

The research tradition in special education makes for a fragile process of decision making. The search for a single perfect study to provide *the* answer is a quixotic quest that has not proved fruitful. As an alternative, the findings from many studies may be combined and integrated in an effort to provide a comprehensive picture about "what the research says." Traditionally, research findings have been combined through either narrative methods providing a verbal report synthesizing individual study findings or numerical methods providing a "box score" tally based on

statistical significance and nonsignificance that presumably identifies the winner. The primary difficulty with these methods is their subjectivity; they lack an explicit, unambiguous, and well-defined context for securing unequivocal outcomes (Jackson, 1980).

Quantitative methods of research synthesis were developed to overcome the perceived difficulties associated with traditional procedures for summarizing research (Glass, 1976). Quantitative methods that have come to be termed meta-analysis involve a process where a number of individual study findings are first rendered comparable with a common metric and then combined statistically to provide answers for the questions of interest (Glass, 1977). The actual techniques of meta-analysis have been comprehensively detailed (e.g., Glass, McGaw, & Smith, 1981) and, although not unequivocally accepted (e.g., Abrami, Cohen, & d'Appolonia, 1988; Slavin, 1984), have become an accepted means of summarizing statistically a research domain (e.g., Cooper & Hedges, 1993; Rosenthal, 1984; Wolf, 1986). The techniques of meta-analysis have also witnessed a number of technical advances (e.g., Bangert-Downs, 1986; Hedges & Olkin, 1985) that have served to enhance objectivity, verifiability, and replicability (Wachter & Straf, 1990).

Meta-analysis is based on a metric termed "effect size" that transforms study data into standard deviation units (*z*-scores). The effect size *(ES)* for studies investigating treatment efficacy is defined by

$$ES = \frac{M_T - M_C}{SD_C}$$

where $M_T$ = mean (average) score of group receiving special intervention, $M_C$ = mean (average) score of comparison (control) group, and $SD_C$ = standard deviation of comparison (control) group.

Individual $ES$ calculations may then be combined and recombined into different aggregations to represent average treatment effects ($\overline{ES}$). The meaning of $ES$ can be translated into notions of overlapping distributions and comparable percentiles. For example, suppose a hypothetical study investigating the efficacy of temporal centripetal therapy revealed an $ES$ of +1.00. The obtained $ES$ of +1.00 indicates an average superiority of one standard deviation for the therapy group. If two separate distributions are drawn for those receiving therapy and those in the control condition, the distributions will be separated by one standard deviation at their means, as shown in Figure 2.

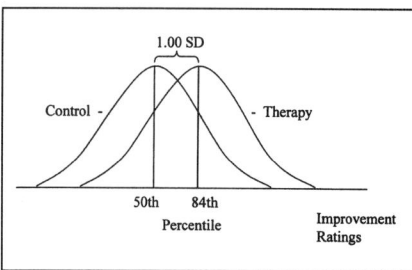

Figure 2. Illustration of the findings from a hypothetical study assessing the efficacy of temporal centripetal therapy.

The average of the therapy curve is located above 84% of the area under the control group curve. This relationship suggests that the student receiving this therapy was better off than 84% of the control group, while only 16% of the control group were left better off than the average student receiving therapy.

Besides notions about distributions and percentiles, it is also possible to offer other interpretations. Cohen (1988), based on notions of statistical power, suggested that $ESs$ may be classified as small (.20), medium (.50), or large (.80). In some cases, $ESs$ are themselves meaningful; zero and negative $ES$ fall into this category. Several other possibilities exist for interpreting $ES$. Comparison might be done within a single meta-analysis. Suppose two special education interventions are compared with traditional instruction: the $ES$ for comparisons of method A and traditional instruction was .50 favoring method A while method B produced an $ES$ of .25 when compared to traditional instruction. Thus, method A was half again more beneficial than method B.

It is also possible to add meaning to $ES$ by reference to known interventions. It is known, for example, that the average student will gain 12 months of achievement over the course of a school year. Thus, the average third-grade student will score 3.0 in early September and 4.0 at the end of the school year. With the known standard deviation of 1.0 grade-equivalent units for most elementary-level standardized achievement tests, the $\overline{ES}$ for one year's instruction at the elementary school level is +1.00. This $\overline{ES}$ can then be used as a basis for comparison. Suppose a new technique (Intervention X) is introduced and the combined $\overline{ES}$ from a number of validation studies is .25. This $\overline{ES}$ is one-fourth as great as the effect of instruction itself (.25 versus 1.00). Hence, Intervention X benefits the average treated subject by the equivalent of one-fourth school year of teaching.

Kavale (1984) described the potential advantages of meta-analysis in terms of enhanced understanding and explanation for special education. By rendering the findings from a number of studies comparable, meta-analysis permits a clarity and explicitness in interpretation that allows conclusions about what the research says. In this volume, for a number of special education interventions and techniques, the extant research is synthesized and placed in context for judging its efficacy. Although the quality of research is an important factor in its review, the meta-analyses reported here do not investigate research quality. The questions surrounding research quality are complex, and the influence of "good" and "poor" research on meta-analytic outcomes subject to debate (see Glass et al., 1981). Rather than dealing with research quality as a variable, the meta-analyses reported do not include discussion of research quality. Research quality was considered in each case, but to provide the most comprehensive analysis, only the very poorest studies were eliminated.

The findings of individual meta-analyses investigating special education practices are presented in subsequent chapters. These analyses examine a range of issues, from explicit intervention techniques to theoretical perspectives underlying intervention approaches. Combined, they offer a basis for judging the effectiveness of special education. Finally, conclusions are drawn about the effectiveness of special education and suggestions offered for making special education more effective.

# CHAPTER 2
# LEARNING ABILITY IN MENTAL RETARDATION

Although students with MR, LD, and E/BD share the common element of school failure, the underlying source of the poor academic achievement may differ. For example, LD historically has been associated with underlying perceptual-motor process deficits that interfere with the learning process. To enhance performance, methods designed to remediate perceptual-motor problems were developed. The work of Kephart (1960), Frostig (see Frostig & Horne, 1964), and Barsch (1967), as examples, focused on particular facets of perceptual-motor functioning with intervention programs developed to remediate the particular perceptual-motor deficits. The goal was to improve the underlying process that was adversely affecting learning and, ultimately, make the learning process more efficient.

In an effort to better understand the learning differences found in students with MR, researchers examined underlying processes related to learning and cognition (e.g., Brooks, Sperber, & McCauley, 1984). The essential paradigm involves comparisons between samples with and without MR on basic laboratory learning tasks as well as experimental strategies designed to enhance learning ability (e.g., Borkowski & Wanschura, 1974; Bray, 1979; Brown, 1974; Cohen, 1983; Evans & Bilsky, 1979; Martin, 1978; Ross & Ward, 1978; Taylor & Turnure, 1979).

The experimental studies have focused on a variety of cognitive deficits associated with MR and on strategies to remediate those deficits. One area of inquiry has involved deficits in discrimi-nation learning where subjects with MR did not attend to relevant task dimensions. A second area focused on memory deficits where subjects with MR were found either to organize input less well or not rehearse material spontaneously in order to embed it in memory. Finally, incidental learning was the focus where subjects with MR have difficulty inhibiting responses to stimuli not the focus of the task or demonstrate a tendency to respond only to certain task dimensions.

## Theoretical Perspectives About Learning Ability in Mental Retardation

The substantial research investigating the various deficits has coalesced into a number of theoretical models explaining the learning process differences associated with MR. To provide perspective, some prominent interpretations are summarized:

*Multiprocess memory theory.* Ellis (1963) originated a stimulus trace theory that was expanded into a multiprocess memory model (Ellis, 1970) incorporating two processes (attention and rehearsal) and three memory stores (primary, secondary, and tertiary). The model suggested that stimuli impress an individual through attention and that information may then be processed for storage in memory. Rehearsal strategies are then used for processing information from primary memory (PM) to secondary memory (SM) or tertiary memory (TM). Information is stored in PM for very short periods before it is forgotten as a result of time or interference. Rehearsal strategies involve a looping process where information is channeled back through PM en route to SM and TM. Retention capabilities are increased as information is transferred from PM to SM to TM in a temporal framework of seconds (PM) to minutes (SM), and finally long-term memory (TM). The primary deficit for individuals with MR involves SM, not PM or TM, and is primarily the result of a failure to use active rehearsal strategies, a failure attributable mainly to inadequate linguistic ability (Ellis, 1970).

*Gestalt organization theory.* Spitz (1963, 1966, 1973a, 1973b) proposed a theoretical position, based in gestalt learning theory, where individuals with MR are deficient in organizing sensory input in a manner meaningful for storage and recall. The learning paradigm is described below.

> When a person learns an item, the process can be broken up in an oversimplified manner as follows:
>
> 1. Browse (person is alert);
>
> 2. Attend (attention is given to specific stimulus);
>
> 3. Input (file into appropriate "hold area");
>
> 4. Recall (return material from temporary file, if necessary);
>
> 5. Storage (put into appropriate permanent file);
>
> 6. Recall (retrieve material from permanent file, if necessary).
>
> Retardates, and normals, may lose information anywhere along the line.... The present paper has emphasized area (3), input, and specifically the organization of the material as it enters for filing. (Spitz, 1966, pp. 52-53)

The theoretical ideas were then presented within a trichotomized schemata of memory. The basic elements were input (stimulus presentation, attention processes, and sensory registration), storage (short- and long-term memory), and retrieval (free recall). It was concluded that "a primary difference between educable retardates and normals is the speed and manner in which retardates scan and selectively organize the material for storage. Chaotic input makes for chaotic retrieval" (Spitz, 1973b, pp. 157-158).

*Attention-retention theory.* Zeaman and House (1963) posited an attention theory of discrimination learning that includes two stages. In the first stage, attention is randomly directed at stimulus dimensions, while, in the second stage, attention is directed primarily at relevant stimulus dimensions. It was found that performance during stage one is a function of intelligence; the lower the MA, the more trials required for performance to improve. For individuals with MR, there is a low probability of attending to relevant stimulus dimensions that significantly slows discrimination learning.

The theory was expanded by Fisher and Zeaman (1973) to include a retention theory that explained how attention deficits may also interfere with retention in short-term memory. Finally, Zeaman and House (1979) elaborated a theory to describe how individuals with MR attend, remember, transfer, extinguish, and ultimately learn.

*Elicitation theory.* Denny (1964, 1966) proposed an elicitation theory to account for the poor incidental learning among individuals with MR. Learning was assumed dependent on the consistent elicitation of to-be-learned responses in close temporal contiguity with particular stimuli. Competing responses that might be elicited by the same or a similar stimulus need to be minimized in order for the requisite learned response to predominate. Because of deficits in attention, linguistic processing, inhibition, and short-term memory, individuals with MR have more difficulty in eliminating competing responses in the presence of cue stimuli.

*Paired-associate learning.* Although more of a specific example than a complete theory, paired-associate learning has been an important source of information on learning ability in individuals with MR. Baumeister (1967) proposed a two-stage model to explain the dynamics of paired-associate learning in individuals with MR. The response stage represents the initial process of association, where the response member of a stimulus-response pair is learned. The associative stage occurs when available responses are associated with their appropriate stimuli. When individuals with MR are taught to use specific cues systematically during the associative stage, their demonstrated performance deficits are minimized.

Baumeister and Kellas (1971) proposed an elaborated model of paired-associate learning where a subject must first decide what is being demanded in the learning task and then select a strategy to deal with the particular task demands. Once coded, the information is stored in memory. Depending on the success of the strategies utilized, a feedback loop is introduced to reinforce responses and ultimately enhance performance.

Each of these theoretical models describing learning deficits in individuals with MR also included suggestions for remediating these deficits and improving learning ability among individuals with MR. Although differing in emphasis and comprehensiveness, the theoretical models have been used as the basis for approaches to remediate learning ability in individuals with MR. For example, several theories suggest that individuals with MR be taught to scan and selectively organize material and to repeat it in organized ways that enhance the potential for later recall. The models described tend to overlap with respect to theoretical concepts and in the nature of the strategies used to enhance learning performance. Nevertheless, research findings about the nature and extent of learning deficits or the relative efficacy of approaches to improving learning performance have demonstrated a variability that makes it difficult to draw definite conclusions.

## Theoretical Models and Remedial Approaches for Learning in Individuals With Mental Retardation

Kavale and Forness (1992) performed a meta-analysis on 268 studies investigating the theoretical and practical implications of the different models describing learning deficits in individuals with MR. The research in question represents a prime example of model-based practice and provides significant insight into the ways theory guides practice. Across 268 studies, 819 *ES* measurements were calculated that represented a total of about 8,000 subjects with a mean age of approximately 15 years, mean IQ of 63, and mean mental age (MA) of 8 years.

## Table 1. Average Effect Size by Theoretical Perspective (Comparison of Subjects With and Without Mental Retardation)

| Theoretical Perspective | Number of Effect Sizes | Mean Effect Size | Percentile Equivalent |
|---|---|---|---|
| Paired-associate learning (Baumeister) | 42 | −.26 | 40 |
| Elicitation theory (Denny) | 22 | −.29 | 39 |
| Multiprocess memory theory (Ellis) | 138 | −.60 | 27 |
| Organizational theory (Spitz) | 161 | −.43 | 34 |
| Attention/retention theory (Zeaman/House) | 58 | −.68 | 25 |
| Other | 20 | −.55 | 29 |
| Unidentified | 102 | −.52 | 30 |

## Comparisons of Subjects With and Without Mental Retardation

The experimental research revealed great diversity with respect to the nature of the tasks used, outcome measures, and research designs. One major difference was related to the nature of the comparison group (individuals with MR vs. individuals without MR). Across 172 studies involving a comparison of subjects with and without MR, the $\overline{ES}$ was −.54, indicating about a one-half SD inferiority for subjects with MR. When compared to subjects without MR who were at the 50th percentile, the average subject with MR was at the 29th percentile, an approximate 21-percentile-rank depressed performance.

To compare and contrast theoretical views, ES data were aggregated by individual theoretical perspective. Two additional categories were included: "other," indicating studies with either close proximity to an existing theoretical model or a less fully developed theoretical view, and "undentified," indicating studies where the rationale and design could not be readily associated with a particular theoretical perspective. The findings are shown in Table 1.

The best performance for subjects with MR was demonstrated in studies using the Baumeister paradigm, where performance was depressed by only 10 percentile ranks (compared to the average 21-percentile-rank depression). Performance at almost the same level was displayed in studies based on Denny's elicitation theory. The poorest performance, on the other hand, was demonstrated by subjects with MR in studies using a Zeaman and House paradigm, where performance was at the 25th percentile of subjects without MR. A similar performance level was found in studies using Ellis's multiprocess memory theory. In these cases, about 75% of subjects without MR outperformed subjects with MR. The subjects with MR performed between the best and worst levels (i.e., 34th percentile) in studies based on Spitz's organizational theory. Both the "other" and "unidentified" classifications revealed the performance of subjects with MR to be closer to the poorest performance levels. Thus, subjects with MR demonstrate learning deficiencies in comparison to subjects without MR, and the magnitude of these differences are related to task variations based on alternative theoretical ideas about the nature of the learning difficulties.

## Task Deficits and Mental Retardation

Each of the theoretical views of MR posits ideas not only about the underlying deficits, but also about the nature of the tasks most adversely affected. The following types of tasks were most often used to investigate the learning deficits of subjects with MR: *Recognition,* correct identification of familiar visual stimuli; *discrimination,* identification among two or more stimuli, one of which is (sometimes arbitrarily) defined as the correct choice; *oddity,* identification, from among (usually three or more) stimuli, of the stimulus differing on a salient dimension; *free recall,* memory for items from among an array of stimuli previously presented; *paired association,* correct matching of a stimulus to its pair from a previously presented set of matched stimuli; *serial learning,* memory for a series of previously presented stimuli in correct order; *memory span,* memory for a series of stimuli in correct order after a brief delay between presentation and recall; *incidental learning,* recall of stimuli not specifically identified as relevant during initial presentation of an array of stimuli; *directed forgetting,* suppression of task dimensions or stimuli, upon recall, that were previously identified or learned as salient; *information processing,* application or use of stimuli previously presented in solving a novel problem; *combination,* two or more of the above

tasks in a single observation; and *other,* tasks not readily identified as one of the above. The data for different task dimensions are presented in Table 2 in descending order (i.e., least to most deficient).

Regardless of task, subjects with MR performed more poorly; in almost 8 out of 10 cases, $\overline{ES}$ s for subjects with MR were negative. Only on tasks involving oddity and incidental learning did subjects with MR approach near average performance levels (i.e., 50th percentile). Performance differences were more pronounced in studies using information processing and "other" tasks. For information processing tasks, the performance of subjects with MR was at the 17th percentile, indicating that they were outperformed by 83% of subjects without MR. The remaining tasks clustered in a narrow range and fell within 5 percentile ranks of each other. On average, when using these tasks, individuals with MR performed at the 30th percentile, indicating they were outperformed by 70% of subjects without MR. When the nature of the task stimuli (e.g., words, letters, digits, pictures, objects, color, forms) was examined, no differences were found.

## Strategy Training and Mental Retardation

The basic deficits demonstrated by subjects with MR on the various tasks represent the fundamental problems interfering with learning. To improve learning ability, a number of strategies have been developed to ameliorate the negative effects of the basic deficits. These strategies included *verbal rehearsal,* repetition of serially presented stimuli, either vocally or subvocally, after initial presentation as a means to enhance recall; *input organization,* systematic ordering or presentation of stimuli to be learned by salient task dimensions; *labeling,* naming stimuli, to be either discriminated or recalled, by salient dimensions during initial presentation; *imagery,* use of visual devices to link together one or more stimuli to enhance subsequent discrimination or recall; *mediation,* use of simple verbal devices to link together stimuli to enhance subsequent discrimination or recall; *verbal elaboration,* use of complex verbal devices to amplify stimuli to enhance subsequent discrimination or recall; *combination,* use of two or more of the above to create a unified strategy; and *other,* strategies not readily identified as one of the above. The data assessing the effectiveness of strategy training on the learning performance of individuals with MR are shown in Table 3 in descending order (i.e., most to least effective).

Across all strategies, the effects of training produced an $\overline{ES}$ of −.50, indicating that the performance of subjects with MR, even with attempts to improve it, remained depressed by approximately 19 percentile ranks, a level about the same as their overall deficit (i.e., depressed by 21 percentile ranks). This suggests little effect for training in terms of relative standing. Thus, almost 70% of subjects without MR still revealed better performance even though subjects with MR were provided with training to enhance performance. In some cases, no strategy training was provided, and these group comparisons produced an $\overline{ES}$ of −.50, which also translates into a 19-percentile-rank inferiority for subjects with MR. This finding suggests that, regardless of whether or not strategy training was implemented, subjects with MR still revealed about the same performance level, and the efficacy of strategy training is called into question.

### Table 2. Average Effect Size by Task Dimension for Subjects With Mental Retardation

| Task Dimension | Number of Effect Sizes | Mean Effect Size | Percentile Equivalent |
|---|---|---|---|
| Oddity | 8 | −.08 | 47 |
| Incidental learning | 27 | −.12 | 45 |
| Combination | 46 | −.34 | 37 |
| Free recall | 89 | −.42 | 34 |
| Paired association | 109 | −.50 | 30 |
| Serial learning | 114 | −.52 | 30 |
| Directed forgetting | 8 | −.54 | 29 |
| Memory span | 25 | −.55 | 29 |
| Recognition | 9 | −.58 | 28 |
| Discrimination | 76 | −.63 | 26 |
| Information processing | 16 | −.95 | 17 |
| Other | 16 | −1.06 | 14 |

With respect to individual strategies, imagery and combination strategies were least effective. Even after training, subjects with MR performed about 30 percentile ranks below average. Falling between the 20th and 30th percentile were three strategies (mediation, other, labeling) where, on average, a subject with MR would show about 27% improvement as a result of strategy training. The remaining strategies (verbal rehearsal, input organization, verbal elaboration) moved subjects with MR above the 30th percentile and appeared to be the most effective in enhancing learning performance.

When investigating strategy use, a common design procedure was to match subjects with MR with comparison subjects on either chronological age (CA) or MA. No differences among strategies were found when comparison was between subjects matched for CA (i.e., MA deficit) versus those matched on MA (i.e., IQ deficit). For groups trained with different strategies, however, differences $\overline{ES}$ among strategies were found, with input organization, rehearsal, and combination strategies tending to be more effective with MA as compared to CA matches. This suggests that some strategy training may attenuate the IQ deficit slightly more than the MA deficit.

## Comparisons With a Control Group With Mental Retardation

The use of subjects without MR as a comparison group can be misleading because, although a strategy may improve performance of both equally, subjects with MR may still remain deficient relative to subjects without MR. To assess this possibility, Table 4 shows the effects of strategy training for subjects with MR compared to control subjects also with MR who received no training. The $\overline{ES}$ data for strategies are presented in descending order (i.e., most effective strategy listed first).

Across all strategies, the $\overline{ES}$ was .70, indicating that the performance of individuals with MR was enhanced by 26 percentile ranks as a result of training. This means that 76% of individuals with

## Table 3. Average Effect Size for Strategy Training (Comparison Group Without Mental Retardation)

| Strategy | Number of Effect Sizes | Mean Effect Size | Percentile Equivalent |
|---|---|---|---|
| Verbal elaboration | 16 | −.40 | 34 |
| Input organization | 130 | −.44 | 33 |
| Verbal rehearsal | 11 | −.46 | 32 |
| Verbal labeling | 3 | −.56 | 29 |
| Other | 37 | −.57 | 28 |
| Mediation | 5 | −.67 | 25 |
| Combination | 20 | −.85 | 20 |
| Imagery | 3 | −.86 | 19 |

## Table 4. Average Effect Size for Strategy Training (Comparison Group With Mental Retardation)

| Strategy | Number of Effect Sizes | Mean Effect Size | Percentile Equivalent |
|---|---|---|---|
| Verbal elaboration | 8 | 1.08 | 86 |
| Mediation | 26 | .98 | 84 |
| Other | 13 | .97 | 83 |
| Imagery | 8 | .92 | 82 |
| Verbal rehearsal | 38 | .67 | 75 |
| Input organization | 55 | .65 | 74 |
| Combination | 43 | .57 | 72 |
| Verbal labeling | 10 | .32 | 63 |

MR demonstrated improved learning ability as a result of training. In some studies where no strategy training was provided, the comparison produced an $\overline{ES}$ of .19, indicating almost no group differences (58th percentile vs. 50th percentile) as opposed to the difference found with training (76th percentile vs. 50th percentile). Thus, with individuals with MR as the control condition as opposed to the case where the comparison group were subjects without MR, strategy training appeared to improve performance across learning tasks.

With respect to individual strategies, all showed positive effects that enhanced performance by anywhere from 8 to 36 percentile ranks. The most effective strategy was verbal elaboration, where 86% of subjects showed enhanced performance. Closely following were the mediation, other, and imagery strategies where, on average, performance was enhanced by 34 percentile ranks. Within 3 percentile ranks of each other were the strategies of input, rehearsal, and combination, where on average individu-

als with MR who received strategy training outperformed 74% of those who did not. The least productive strategy was verbal labeling, where the gain from training was 13 percentile ranks, compared to 36 percentile ranks for the most productive, verbal elaboration).

Two factors appeared to influence the efficacy of strategy training. The first was length of training (i.e., on one day for either a fixed session or to criterion over several sessions, 2–4 days, one week, greater than one week) where the greater-than-one-week $\overline{ES}$ of 1.35 was significantly larger than the other three training periods, with $\overline{ES}$ of .43 (on one day for a fixed session or to criterion over several sessions), .64 (2–4 days), and .59 (one week). The second factor was intelligence; subjects with borderline intellectual function (IQ above 70 but below 85) improved more than subjects with mild mental retardation (IQ 50–70) who in turn improved more than subjects with severe mental retardation (IQ below 50), as revealed by $\overline{ES}$ of 1.5, .63, and .02, respectively.

# Conclusion

The most general conclusion to be drawn from these analyses is that the performance of subjects with MR was inferior to that of subjects without MR across theoretical perspectives, task dimensions, learning strategies, and comparisons (CA and MA). Although not unexpected, the findings are difficult to generalize to current special education programs for two reasons. First, fewer than 1 in 8 subjects were below the moderate range of MR, while some subjects would no longer quality for the MR category because of IQ levels above the current cut-off of 70 or 75. Second, most studies included in the analysis were more than 25 years old; the average publication date was 1970. Although this was a fairly recent meta-analysis, it is clear that very few studies of strategy training with MR samples have been completed in recent years despite the potential importance of this work for classroom teachers. Within this context, it is also important to note that the field of MR has undergone significant change, most notably in the form of a population that is declining in numbers and showing a fundamentally different nature (MacMillan & Forness, 1993; Polloway & Smith, 1988).

With these limitations, it is difficult to place the one-half SD performance deficit of subjects with MR in context. Only on information processing tasks were the deficits particularly marked. Additionally, the hypothesis that serial learning tasks would be more difficult than paired-associate learning for some individuals with MR (e.g., Jensen, 1970) was not supported. Both tasks were widely studied but showed remarkably similar findings (see Table 2). In instructing students with MR, practitioners have traditionally been encouraged to avoid having some students learn a series of items in favor of pairing items to be learned with already familiar items. The present findings, at least, question whether preference for one strategy over another is always warranted. This conclusion is underscored by the finding that serial learning tended to be significantly enhanced by strategy training, especially in CA-matched subjects.

A notable finding is that in comparisons with both MR and non-MR control groups, strategy training improved learning performance but produced no change in relative standing of subjects with MR, whose performance remained deficient even after training. Previously, there has been an optimistic view about attenuating learning deficits associated with MR through systematic strategy training. The deficits in question appear real and, even after training, continued to place students with MR at a disadvantage in classroom learning. This is not to suggest training is inconsequential; subjects with MR who received strategy training improved their learning abilities substantially more than subjects who received no such training (see Table 4). Additionally, with the exception of verbal labeling, a variety of strategies revealed positive results (i.e., about a one-SD advantage over controls) and, consequently, contribute to enhanced learning ability.

Across both comparison groups (i.e., controls with and without MR), strategy training tended to bring less benefit to those with moderate or severe levels of MR. There was also a "younger-the-better" trend when subjects with MR were compared to subjects without MR, and a "longer-the-better" trend when subjects with MR were compared to their counterparts receiving no training. This latter finding suggests that a single lesson "quick fix" may not produce gains that are as sustainable as those produced by a week or more of strategy training. Altogether, these findings question the malleability of learning deficits for individuals with moderate-to-severe MR.

The studies included in the present meta-analysis had to meet relatively strict inclusion criteria (e.g., be theoretically based, conducted in a laboratory setting, focused on specific learning deficits). The perceived decline in such studies over the years may not reflect actual research efforts in the area, particularly if the interest is in, for example, investigating more ecologically relevant strategies or strategies not reflecting a specific theoretical perspective. Nonetheless, the present findings serve to highlight concerns expressed about declining research interest in mild MR. There is an argument that much of the research may be irrelevant to instruction because of its limited applicability to classroom learning (e.g., Brooks & Baumeister, 1977; Forness, 1981; MacMillan & Meyers, 1984). Classroom instruction is viewed as far too complex to be captured in laboratory studies testing theoretical models, because they seek to isolate and control only one or two research variables. The complex dynamics of the classroom are not captured, and it becomes difficult to determine whether the theoretical implications for practice are effective in the "real world." Still another argument questions the wisdom of "remediating" specific cognitive abilities of individuals with MR as opposed to more intense

preparation for settings beyond school (e.g., Kramer, Piersel, & Glover, 1988; Patton, Cronin, Polloway, Hutchinson, & Robinson, 1989; Polloway, Patton, Smith, & Roderique, 1992). A final argument links the decline of research in mild MR with a decline in the number of individuals being identified in the MR category (Forness & Kavale, 1984; MacMillan, 1989; Polloway & Smith, 1988). As a consequence, the research base is seriously compromised because assumptions about learning deficits in MR have been based largely on studies that focus on a population no longer identified as eligible for the MR category. Additionally, it has been argued that research on more severe levels of MR should be a priority because of the more evident needs of individuals in this group (Berkson & Landesman-Dwyer, 1977).

Given these constraints, the present findings need to be placed in context. It seems safe to conclude that, for individuals with MR, strategy training that directly addresses deficits in learning ability produces benefits. Although there is limited improvement in the relative standing of individuals with MR compared to individuals without MR as a result of strategy training, their relative performance over peers with MR but without strategy training suggests substantial improvement. The difficulty, however, is that many of the individuals with MR who are comparable to the original subjects in which these findings were established may no longer be eligible for such strategy training because they are now ineligible for special education.

# CHAPTER 3
# PROCESS TRAINING

Process training possesses a long and glorious history in special education; in fact, process training represents one of the oldest forms of general education (see Mann, 1979). Although the theoretical ideas presented in chapter 2 were used to design intervention approaches specifically for individuals with MR, process training was initially formulated for all special education groups. The goal was to design activities that might enhance all processes assumed to underlie learning ability and thus improve learning performance. With the creation of the category of learning disabilities, process training reached its zenith as a popular intervention for special education.

Process training has taken a variety of forms, and whether the goal has been to train processes, abilities, powers, potentials, factors, capacities, or faculties, the idea has been to enhance these functions to ultimately improve learning performance. At the same time, however, there has been debate about process training. For example, fundamental questions about the nature of processes have been raised: Are processes merely hypothetical constructs or are they substantive realities? Besides theoretical debate about process concepts, the effectiveness of process training programs has been subject to long-standing debate. Although the question of efficacy is still open, process training has always possessed a powerful intuitive appeal captured in the assumption that what is most fundamental is training the mind and its processes (powers, abilities, capacities, faculties), even at the expense of direct instruction in basic skill areas.

This "was what Socrates and Plato said and what Itard, Seguin, Montessori, and Binet reiterated. It is what the Frostigs, Kirks, Kepharts, seem to have been saying more recently" (Mann, 1979, p. 537).

With special education continually called upon to answer what is special about itself, methods like process training were likened to rain upon parched land; this "new scientific pedagogy was going to revitalize education, provide individual prescriptive correctives for learning problems, reclaim the cognitively impaired" (Mann, 1979, p. 538). Regardless of its intuitive appeal, process training has not received unequivocal empirical support. Process training has been supported more on metaphysical grounds than through empirical evidence. This has led to long-standing debate about the effectiveness of process training. What does the empirical evidence show? Are less equivocal conclusions possible? The findings from three meta-analyses investigating these questions with regard to perceptual-motor, psycholinguistic, and modality training follow.

## Perceptual-Motor Training

The most popular forms of process training in special education have been programs that attempt to mitigate perceptual-motor deficits that were assumed to be the basic problem experienced by individuals with learning disabilities. A number of clinical reports have attested to the efficacy of perceptual-motor training and popularized it as a favored intervention for learning disabilities (e.g., Arena, 1969; Barsch,

1967; Van Witsen, 1967). Besides these positive clinical reports, experimental studies have tested the validity of perceptual-motor interventions and have been reviewed selectively (e.g., Balow, 1971; Footlik, 1971; Goodman & Hammill, 1973; Hammill, Goodman, & Wiederholt, 1974). Although the conclusions drawn generally did not favor perceptual-motor training, caution was urged because the research studies were marked by faulty reporting and questionable methodological practices. In addition, philosophical attacks on perceptual-motor training appeared (Mann, 1970, 1971a), but their validity was challenged (Kephart, 1972). Thus, the efficacy of perceptual-motor training was fertile ground for a quantitative synthesis that could attempt to bring closure to a disparate literature.

Kavale and Mattson (1983) found 180 experiments assessing the efficacy of perceptual-motor training that produced a total of 637 $ES$ measurements. The studies represented about 13,000 subjects whose average age was 8 years and average IQ was 89; they had received an average of 65 hours of perceptual-motor training. The $\overline{ES}$ across 637 $ES$ measurements was .08, which, in relative terms, indicates that a student no better off than average (i.e., at the 50th percentile), rises to the 53rd percentile as a result of perceptual-motor interventions. At the end of treatment, the average trained subject was better off than 53% of control subjects, a gain only slightly better than no treatment at all (50%). Additionally, of 637 $ES$ measurements, 48% were negative, suggesting that the probability of obtaining a positive response to training was only slightly better than chance.

The effects of perceptual-motor training appear to be negligible, but a single index assessing efficacy may mask particular situations where perceptual-motor training might be more effective. Consequently, $ES$ data were aggregated into increasingly differentiated outcome groupings, and the findings are shown in Tables 5, 6, and 7.

The findings speak for themselves: Regardless of how global or discrete the aggregation, perceptual-motor training provides no evidence of effectiveness. There were few positive effects and no indications suggesting an effective intervention.

Tables 8 and 9 provide aggregated $ES$ data for special education category and grade level. Interpretation is unencumbered: Essentially zero effects are seen for all classifications and at all grade levels. These data suggest that there are no selected benefits for perceptual-motor training; in no instance was perceptual-motor intervention effective.

Perceptual-motor training programs have taken a variety of forms, and the associated names read like the roster from a special education hall of fame. The $\overline{ES}$s for the various training methods are shown in Table 10. The findings are not encouraging: There is no indication of positive effects. Studies investigating the efficacy of individual programs included research performed by both independent investigators and program advocates, and an example will reveal the fragility that may be associated with such research findings. The Delacato program (e.g., Delacato, 1959), based upon the concept of neurological patterning, was assessed by both Delacato disciples (see Delacato, 1966) and more critical investigators (e.g., Cohen, Birch, & Taft, 1970; Glass & Robbins, 1967). The Delacato sources produced an $\overline{ES}$ of .72 and the non-Delacato sources revealed an $\overline{ES}$ of −.24.

## Table 5. Average Effect Size for Perceptual-Motor Outcome Classes

| Outcome Class | Number of Effect Sizes | Mean Effect Size | Percentile Equivalent |
|---|---|---|---|
| Perceptual/Sensory motor | 233 | .17 | 58 |
| Academic achievement | 283 | .01 | 50 |
| Cognitive/Aptitude | 95 | .03 | 51 |
| Adaptive behavior | 26 | .27 | 61 |

## Table 6. Average Effect Size for Perceptual-Motor General Outcome Categories

| General Outcome Category | Number of Effect Sizes | Mean Effect Size | Percentile Equivalent |
|---|---|---|---|
| *Perceptual/Sensory motor* | | | |
| Gross motor | 44 | .21 | 58 |
| Fine motor | 28 | .18 | 57 |
| Visual perception | 145 | .15 | 56 |
| Auditory perception | 16 | .12 | 55 |
| *Academic achievement* | | | |
| Arithmetic | 26 | .10 | 54 |
| Readiness | 69 | .08 | 53 |
| Handwriting | 12 | .05 | 52 |
| Language | 18 | .03 | 51 |
| Spelling | 16 | .02 | 51 |
| Reading | 142 | −.04 | 48 |
| *Cognitive/Aptitude* | | | |
| Performance IQ | 34 | .07 | 53 |
| Verbal IQ | 53 | −.01 | 50 |

## Table 7. Average Effect Size for
## Perceptual-Motor Specific Outcome Categories

| Specific Outcome Category | Number of Effect Sizes | Mean Effect Size | Percentile Equivalent |
|---|---|---|---|
| *Gross motor skills* | | | |
| Body awareness/image | 22 | .26 | 60 |
| Balance/posture | 14 | .26 | 60 |
| Locomotor skills | 8 | −.02 | 49 |
| *Visual perceptual skills* | | | |
| Visual-motor ability | 26 | .22 | 59 |
| Figure-ground discrimination | 28 | .17 | 57 |
| Visual discrimination | 31 | .15 | 56 |
| Visual spatial perception | 16 | .14 | 56 |
| Visual integration | 17 | .09 | 54 |
| Visual memory | 15 | .06 | 52 |
| *Reading achievement* | | | |
| Vocabulary | 25 | −.01 | 50 |
| Word recognition | 36 | −.02 | 49 |
| Oral reading | 17 | −.04 | 48 |
| Speed/rate | 8 | −.04 | 48 |
| Comprehension | 33 | −.06 | 48 |

## Table 8. Average Effect Size for
## Subject Groups Receiving Perceptual-Motor Training

| General Outcome Categories | Number of Effect Sizes | Mean Effect Size | Percentile Equivalent |
|---|---|---|---|
| Moderately mentally retarded (IQ = 25–50) | 66 | .15 | 55 |
| Mildly mentally retarded (IQ = 50–75) | 143 | .13 | 55 |
| Motor disabled | 118 | .12 | 55 |
| Slow learner (IQ = 75–90) | 14 | .10 | 54 |
| General education | 58 | .05 | 52 |
| Learning disabled | 77 | .02 | 51 |
| Reading disabled | 74 | −.01 | 50 |

## Table 9. Average Effect Size by Grade Level for Perceptual-Motor Training

| Grade Level | Number of Effect Sizes | Mean Effect Size | Percentile Equivalent |
|---|---|---|---|
| Preschool | 47 | .05 | 52 |
| Kindergarten | 129 | .10 | 54 |
| Primary elementary (grades 1–3) | 226 | .08 | 53 |
| Middle elementary (grades 4–6) | 74 | .07 | 53 |
| Junior high school | 67 | .09 | 54 |
| High school | 67 | .09 | 54 |

## Table 10. Average Effect Size for Perceptual-Motor Training Programs

| Training Program | Number of Effect Sizes | Mean Effect Size | Percentile Equivalent |
|---|---|---|---|
| Barsch (1967) Movigenic training | 18 | .16 | 56 |
| Cratty (1969) Perceptual-motor training | 27 | .11 | 54 |
| Delacato (1959) Neurological patterning | 79 | .16 | 56 |
| Frostig (1964) Visual-perceptual training | 173 | .10 | 54 |
| Getman (1965) Visuomotor training | 48 | .12 | 55 |
| Kephart (1960) Perceptual-motor training | 132 | .06 | 52 |

A nonselective and uncritical interpretation of these studies could thus result in very different conclusions.

The findings from this meta-analysis would support the position statement offered by the Council for Learning Disabilities (CLD) where they suggested

There is little or no empirical support for claims that the training of perceptual and perceptual-motor functions improves either academic performance or perceptual or perceptual-motor functions… schools must view the time, money, and other resources devoted to such activities as wasteful, as an obstruction to provision of appropriate services, and as unwarranted for any purposes other than those of pure research. (CLD, 1986, p. 247)

Yet, there have been suggestions that the available evidence does not permit either a positive or negative evaluation of perceptual-motor training (e.g., Hallahan & Cruickshank, 1973). The quantitative synthesis presented here found no significant benefits and appears to provide the negative evaluation necessary for questioning the value of perceptual-motor training. The empirical evidence seems unequivocal but must face the challenge presented by the deep historical roots and positive clinical tradition attesting to the efficacy of perceptual-motor training.

# Psycholinguistic Training

Psycholinguistic training represents another type of process training that, at one time, was among the most popular special education interventions. Training was based on test findings from the once popular Illinois Test of Psycholinguistic Abilities (ITPA) (Kirk, McCarthy, & Kirk, 1968), which assessed receptive, integrative, and expressive abilities by presenting stimuli in auditory and visual channels. Test findings were assumed to reveal intraindividual deficits that would then be subjected to treatment through a variety of remedial and developmental programs.

Psycholinguistic training is based on the assumption that discrete psychological and linguistic abilities can be identified and trained. The assumption about training touched off a long-standing debate that represented very different philosophical perspectives about the nature of special education interventions. A number of research studies were undertaken and were reviewed periodically, but interpretation showed significant differences, and decisions about the effectiveness of psycholinguistic training became increasingly difficult.

In a 1974 review, Hammill and Larsen summarized the findings from 39 studies in terms of statistical significance or non-significance. They constructed a table with either a "+" (significant) or "0" (nonsignificant) for total ITPA score, ITPA subtests, or both. This vote-counting methodology led them to conclude that

"researchers have been unsuccessful in developing those skills which would enable their subjects to do well on ITPA…[and]…the idea that psycholinguistic constructs, as measured by ITPA, can be trained by existing techniques remains nonvalidated" (Hammill & Larsen, 1974, p. 10-11).

Minskoff (1975) offered a critique of Hammill and Larsen's (1974) review:

> Because of Hammill and Larsen's oversimplified approach, 39 studies with noncomparable subjects and treatments were grouped together. Moreover, for the most part, they reviewed methodologically inadequate studies in which there was short term training using general approaches to treatment primarily with mentally retarded or disadvantaged subjects having no diagnosed learning disabilities. (Minskoff, 1975, p. 137)

In effect, Minskoff suggested that Hammill and Larsen had compared "apples and oranges," and 10 specific methodological errors were described. Minskoff suggested that psycholinguistic deficits can respond to training, and concluded by decrying the skepticism surrounding psycholinguistic training, saying, "It can be dangerous if it leads to the abolition of training methods that may be beneficial to some children with psycholinguistic disabilities" (p. 143).

Immediately following was a response by Newcomer, Larsen, and Hammill (1975) that contested the major points made by Minskoff (1975). Suffice it to say that the rhetoric became increasingly confusing and enmeshed in trivial controversy. Nevertheless, Newcomer et al. contended that "the reported literature raises doubts regarding the efficacy of presently available Kirk-Osgood psycholinguistic training programs" (p. 147).

The debate lay dormant for some 3 years when Lund, Foster, and McCall-Perez (1978) offered a reevaluation of the 39 studies analyzed by Hammill and Larsen (1974). The studies were reexamined individually to determine the validity of negative conclusions regarding the effectiveness of psycholinguistic training. Of the 24 studies, 6 clearly showed positive results for psycholinguistic training and "contraindicate the conclusions that such training is nonvalidated" (Lund et al., 1978, p. 317). Of 10 studies showing negative results, only 2 were reported accurately; the remaining 8 were either equivocal or showed positive results. Lund et al. reached conclusions markedly at variance with the statement that psycholinguistic training has not been validated:

> Our analysis indicates that some studies show significant positive results as measured by ITPA, some studies show positive results in the areas remediated, and some do not show results from which any conclusions can be drawn. It is, therefore, not logical to conclude either that all studies in psycholinguistic training are effective or that all studies in psycholinguistic training are not effective. (Lund et al., 1978, p. 317)

The special education community did not wait long for the debate to continue. Hammill and Larsen (1978) reaffirmed their original position.

> The cumulative results of the pertinent research have failed to demonstrate that psycholinguistic training has value, at least with the ITPA as the criterion for successful training. It is

important to note that, regardless of the reevaluations by propsycholinguistic educators, the current state of the research strongly questions the efficacy of psycholinguistic training and suggests that programs designed to improve psycholinguistic functioning need to be viewed cautiously and monitored with great care. (p. 413)

After some 5 years of debate, polemics abounded but a nagging question remained: What is really known about the efficacy of psycholinguistic training? In an effort to bring closure, Kavale (1981) performed a meta-analysis on 34 studies investigating the effectiveness of psycholinguistic training. The 34 studies yielded 240 $ESs$ that produced an $\overline{ES}$ of .39. This finding was based on data representing approximately 1,850 subjects who averaged 7.5 years of age with a mean IQ of 82. They had received an average of 50 hours of psycholinguistic training. Thus, the average subject receiving psycholinguistic training stands at approximately the 65th percentile of subjects receiving no special psycholinguistic training; the latter remain at the 50th percentile. Table 11 presents $\overline{ES}$s classified by ITPA subtest.

Five of the 10 regularly administered ITPA subtests show small, albeit positive, effects; it is questionable, however, whether these psycholinguistic abilities respond to training and whether they should be subjected to training. The case is different for four subtests: Auditory and Visual Association, Verbal and Manual Expression. For these psycholinguistic abilities, training improves functioning from 15 to 24 percentile ranks. Thus, the average trained subject would be better off than approximately 65% to 74% of untrained subjects with respect to associative and expressive abilities.

27

## Table 11.  Average Effect Size for Psycholinguistic Training by Illinois Test of Psycholinguistic Abilities (ITPA) Subtest

| ITPA Subtest | Number of Effect Sizes | Mean Effect Size | Percentile Equivalent |
|---|---|---|---|
| Auditory reception | 20 | .21 | 58 |
| Visual reception | 20 | .21 | 58 |
| Auditory association | 24 | .44 | 67 |
| Visual association | 21 | .39 | 65 |
| Verbal expression | 24 | .63 | 74 |
| Manual expression | 23 | .54 | 71 |
| Grammatic closure | 21 | .30 | 62 |
| Visual closure | 5 | .48 | 68 |
| Auditory sequential memory | 21 | .32 | 63 |
| Visual sequential memory | 21 | .27 | 61 |
| *Supplementary subtests* | | | |
| Auditory closure | 3 | −.05 | 48 |
| Sound blending | 3 | .38 | 65 |

Subtests of the ITPA were patterned upon psycholinguistic constructs derived from dimensions of Osgood's (1957) model of communication. Table 12 presents an analysis of the effects of training upon the theoretical psycholinguistic dimensions and their constructs underlying the ITPA.

Expressive Processes showed the greatest response to psycholinguistic training, while small effects were noted for Receptive Processes and at the Automatic Level. The analysis offered by Hammill and Larsen (1974) suggested that both Representational Level and the Visual-Motor Modality were not particularly responsive to training, but the obtained $\overline{ES}$s of .40 and .38 respectively for these abilities belie such an interpretation. Consequently, the 16- and 15-percentile-rank improvement shown by trained subjects for Representational Level and Visual-Motor Modalities cannot be easily dismissed.

The *ES* data were next integrated by approach and method for psycholinguistic training, and the findings are shown in Table 13.

Not surprisingly, prescriptive/individualized approaches were found superior to generalized/nonindividualized methods. As with many other educational approaches, individualized instruction proved superior. The next finding was surprising: The *Peabody Language Development Kits* (PLDK) (Dunn & Smith, 1967) demonstrated the largest $\overline{ES}$ when compared to both ITPA-related activities and other methods (e.g., sensory, perceptual, or motor training activities).

## Table 12. Average Effect Size for Psycholinguistic Training by Illinois Test of Psycholinguistic Abilities (ITPA) Construct

| ITPA Dimension | Construct | Number of Effect Sizes | Mean Effect Size | Percentile Equivalent |
|---|---|---|---|---|
| Level | Representational | 132 | 40 | 66 |
| | Automatic | 68 | .21 | 58 |
| | ProcessReception | 40 | .21 | 58 |
| | Organization | 119 | .32 | 63 |
| | Expression | 47 | .59 | 72 |
| Modality | Auditory-Verbal | 110 | .32 | 63 |
| | Visual-Motor | 90 | .38 | 65 |

## Table 13. Average Effect Size for Psycholinguistic Training by Study Features

| Feature | Number of Effect Sizes | Mean Effect Size | Percentile Equivalent |
|---|---|---|---|
| *Approach* | | | |
| General/Nonindividualized | 38 | .37 | 64 |
| Prescriptive/Individualized | 6 | .49 | 69 |
| *Method* | | | |
| Activities based on the ITPA[a] | 12 | .30 | 62 |
| Peabody language systems[b] | 14 | .49 | 69 |
| Other[c] | 9 | .35 | 64 |

[a]Illinois Test of Psycholinguistic Abilities. [b]Peabody Language Development Kit. [c]Sensory, motor, or perceptual training activities.

On the surface, the superiority of the PLDK appears contrary to expectation, because ITPA-type activities should be most closely related to the criterion measure, the ITPA itself. Upon reflection, these findings are not surprising if viewed in terms of program structure. The PLDK represents a highly structured sequence of lessons designed to enhance general verbal ability. Although many ITPA training procedures are based on the Osgood-Kirk model (e.g., Bush & Giles, 1977; Kirk & Kirk, 1971), they are only suggestions and guidelines for training activities and do not provide sequential, structured activities like those in the PLDK. Consequently, they do not represent a comprehensive training package but merely examples for psycholinguistic training activities that must be structured and planned by individual teachers (Kavale, 1982b).

The present findings appear to provide a cautious but affirmative answer to the question of the effectiveness of psycho-linguistic training. In particular instances, psycholinguistic training demonstrated positive outcomes and cast doubt on previous conclusions such as "the overwhelming consensus of research evidence concerning the effectiveness of psycholinguistic training is that it remains essentially nonvalidated" (Hammill & Larsen, 1978, p. 412). Hammill and Larsen (1974) probably overstated their case when they concluded that "neither the ITPA subtests nor their theoretical constructs are particularly ameliorative" (p. 12). Clearly, the findings regarding the benefits of intervention for the Expressive processes, particularly Verbal Expression, and subtests at the Representational Level are encouraging: They embody the "linguistic" aspects of the ITPA and, ultimately, productive language behavior.

These findings, however, only fueled the debate over the efficacy of psycholinguistic training. Larsen, Parker, and Hammill (1982), for example, suggested that Kavale (1981) had reviewed a body of literature that was more favorable to psycholinguistic training and thus different from that used by Hammill and Larsen (1974). Upon analysis, however, the difference amounted to four studies that would have added 28 $ES$ measurements to the 240 obtained and would have led to an overall decline in $\overline{ES}$ of .04, on average, across subtests. This $\overline{ES}$ decline, from .39 to .35, means that instead of 65% of students receiving psycholinguistic training being better off than a control group, 64% would now be better off; this is an inconsequential decline and does not qualify the finding as an inflated estimate.

For a basic area like language, after a year of schooling, the average elementary school student has gained about one standard deviation ($\overline{ES} = +1.00$) and exceeds about 84% of scores made on a language achievement measure at the beginning of the school year. The approximately 60% success rate for training Verbal Expression is thus substantial. In fact, roughly 50 hours of psycholinguistic training produced benefits on the ITPA Verbal Expression subtest ($\overline{ES} = .63$), exceeding that which would be expected from one-half year of instruction in language ($\overline{ES} = .50$).

Larsen et al. (1982) as well as Sternberg and Taylor (1982) questioned the findings on a cost-benefit basis since the gains represented only about 15–20 items across ITPA subtests. A distinction was made between statistical significance and practical significance, with Sternberg and Taylor (1982) pursuing the question, "Does the increase of only two or three items per subtest within this instrument really make a *clinically significant* difference?" (p. 255).

The answer is affirmative, and the example of Verbal Expression demonstrates why. In concrete terms, the obtained training effect for Verbal Expression ($\overline{ES} = .63$) translates into improvement by perhaps an additional half-dozen correct responses on the ITPA. If these six items are considered proxies for hundreds of language skills and abilities, then improvement on these seemingly few items is significant. Consider an analogous situation: A student with IQ 130 answers perhaps nine more Information questions or nine more Vocabulary items on the Wechsler than a student with IQ 100. Does this suggest that the difference between IQ 100 and IQ 130 is represented by these nine bits of knowledge? Certainly, the underlying abilities involved transcend nine pieces of information or words. Likewise, improvement on the Verbal Expression subtest represents more than the expected increase of six test items because it comprises a complex amalgam of language abilities. Thus, for a student deficient in the areas enhanced by psycholinguistic training, a remedial program is likely to provide salutary effects and advantages for the student that probably surpass the particular subtests themselves.

## Modality Training

The practice of assessing individual abilities and devising subsequent instruction in accord with assessed ability patterns possesses a long history and intuitive appeal (e.g., Dunn, 1979). Whether it is termed the modality model, learning styles, aptitude x treatment interaction, differential programming, or diagnostic-prescriptive teaching, the benefits are widely believed (e.g., Dunn & Dunn, 1978) even though the weight of the evidence has not been supportive (e.g., Cronbach & Snow, 1977). Its deep historical roots and strong clinical support have prevented the modality model from being questioned as a validated special education practice (see

Carbo, 1983). Arter and Jenkins (1977), for example, found that 99% of teachers surveyed believed that a student's modality strengths and weaknesses should be considered and that a student learned more when instruction was modified to match preferred modality patterns.

Kavale and Forness (1987) synthesized data from 39 studies evaluating the modality model (i.e., assessing modality preferences and matching instruction to those preferences). The 39 studies yielded 318 *ES* measurements and represented about 3,100 subjects whose average age was 8.66 years and average IQ was 98. Because the modality model includes two components, testing and teaching, no substantive insight is provided by a single index.

On the assessment side, the *ES* measurements indicate the level of differentiation between subjects chosen because of assessed modal preferences and those demonstrating no such preferences. A total of 113 *ES* measurements examined the assessment of modality preferences and the findings are shown in Table 14.

The first $\overline{ES}$ column represents the magnitude of group differentiation as originally calculated. The tests used to assess modality preferences have been

### Table 14. Average Effect Size for Modality Assessments

| Modality | Number of Effect Sizes | Mean Effect Size (Uncorrected) | Mean Effect Size (Corrected) | % of Subjects Differentiated From Comparison Group |
|---|---|---|---|---|
| Auditory | 47 | .93 | .55 | 71 |
| Visual | 46 | .90 | .51 | 70 |
| Kinesthetic | 20 | .97 | .43 | 67 |

shown to possess poor reliabilities (see Ysseldyke & Salvia, 1980), and this suggests that these *ES* measurements need to be corrected for the influence of measurement error in order to provide a "true" level of group differentiation (see Hunter, Schmidt, & Jackson, 1982).

Across the 113 *ES* measurements, for example, the $\overline{ES}$, after correction, declined from .93 to .51; on average, 70% of subjects demonstrating a modality preference could be differentiated clearly on the basis of their test scores while 30% could not be distinguished unequivocally. With the original $\overline{ES}$ (.93), the one standard deviation (*SD*) difference typically used as a criterion to establish modality group membership was approached but, after correction for measurement error, only 7 out of 10 subjects actually demonstrated a modality preference score different enough to warrant placement in a particular modality preference group, while 3 out of 10 would be misplaced in a modality preference group.

Although modality assessments were presumed to differentiate subjects with respect to modality preferences, there was, in actuality, considerable overlap between preference and nonpreference groups. Much of the difficulty was the result of test unreliability and, when *ES* was corrected for test unreliability, it was found that measurement error reduced the distinction among modality groups to a level no better than, on average, 2 out of 3 correct placement decisions.

Besides assessing modality preferences, the 39 studies also evaluated the effect of matching instruction to preferred modalities. Of the 318 *ES* measurements, 205 assessed the effectiveness of modality teaching; these findings are displayed in Table 15.

The 205 *ES* measurements produced an $\overline{ES}$ of .14, which translates into only a 6-percentile-rank improvement and indicates that 56% of experimental subjects were better off after modality instruction. This result is only slightly above chance (50%) and indicates conversely that 44% of experimental subjects did not reveal any gain from modality-matched instruction. Furthermore, 72 *ES* measurements (35%) were negative, indicating that over one-third of subjects receiving instruction matched to their preferred learning modality actually scored less well than comparison subjects receiving no special modality-based instruction.

Within the achievement domain, reading was a primary area where the effects of modality-matched instruction were evaluated. Reading achievement data are displayed in Table 16. Across modalities, modality-matched instruction produced gains from 2 (comprehension) to 7 (vocabulary and spelling) percentile ranks; these levels of improvement are small. Only 57% of experimental subjects would show benefits from modality-based instruction, while 43% would not. Modality teaching appears to have only modest effects on improving reading abilities. When instructional methods were matched to modality preferences, the positive effects were also small. Across reading skills, 38% (6 out of 16) of the comparisons in Table 16 revealed modality teaching effects that were not different from zero (as shown by a 95% confidence interval).

In providing answers to the question "Why teach through modality strengths?" Barbe and Milone (1981) suggested that research supported the contention that modality-based instruction works. Although the presumption of matching

## Table 15. Average Effect Size for Modality-Matched Instruction

| Modality | Number of Effect Sizes | Mean Effect Size | Percentile Equivalent |
|---|---|---|---|
| Auditory | 80 | .18 | 57 |
| Visual | 81 | .09 | 54 |
| Kinesthetic | 44 | .18 | 57 |

## Table 16. Average Effect Size for Modality-Matched Instruction on Reading Skills

| | Modality | | | | | | | | | | |
|---|---|---|---|---|---|---|---|---|---|---|---|
| | Total | | | Auditory | | | Visual | | | Kinesthetic | | |
| Skill | $n$ | $\overline{ES}$ | % | $n$ | $\overline{ES}$ | % | $n$ | $\overline{ES}$ | % | $n$ | $\overline{ES}$ | % |
| Word recognition | 75 | .15 | 56 | 28 | .20 | 58 | 33 | .08 | 53 | 14 | .20 | 58 |
| Comprehension | 38 | .05 | 52 | 15 | .06 | 52 | 16 | .03 | 51 | 7 | .04 | 52 |
| Vocabulary | 45 | .17 | 57 | 18 | .19 | 58 | 17 | .14 | 56 | 10 | .19 | 58 |
| Spelling | 47 | .18 | 57 | 19 | .25 | 60 | 15 | .09 | 54 | 13 | .22 | 59 |

Note. $n$ = number of effect sizes. $\overline{ES}$ = mean effect size. % = percentile equivalent.

instructional strategies to individual modality preferences to enhance learning efficiency possesses great intuitive appeal, little empirical support for this proposition was found. With respect to modality assessment, it was shown that groups seemingly differentiated on the basis of modality preferences actually revealed considerable overlap, and it was doubtful whether any of the presumed preferences could really be deemed preferences. On the teaching side, little (or no) gain in achievement was found when instructional methods were matched to preferred learning modality.

The present negative findings contravene the conventional wisdom found in statements such as these:

All children do not learn the same way. They rely on different sensory modes to help them. Some depend heavily on their sense of sight, others on their sense of hearing, and still others on their sense of touch. The mode they use influences their classroom behavior and achievement. (Barbe & Milone, 1980, p. 45)

The negative evaluation of the modality model by Kavale and Forness (1987) did not go unchallenged. Dunn (1990) suggested that the conclusions were biased and were based on inappropriate choices. The bias was related to the presumption that the studies chosen suffered from serious design flaws. Additionally, the fact that most studies used standardized tests to measure outcomes was considered a liability rather than an asset. With respect to inappropriate choices, it was suggested that Kavale and Forness did not take into account presumed modality differences between younger and older students; the multiplicity among preference patterns, suggesting that individual modalities cannot be studied in isolation; the proper definition and interpretation of the terms auditory, visual, and kinesthetic with regard to modality; and instrumentation problems preventing valid measurement of the constructs.

Dunn (1990) then challenged the interpretation of $\overline{ES}$ by suggesting that because the samples studied were students with disabilities, any positive findings should be considered laudatory; in addition, because of the difficulties in attaining achievement gains on standardized tests, even the modest gains demonstrated were excellent and might be unusual in general education. Dunn presented findings from 10 studies that presumably overcame the difficulties cited and revealed significantly higher achievement for students taught through modality preferences.

Kavale and Forness (1990) responded to Dunn's (1990) critique, and the specifics are not important. Of greater importance were difficulties involved in judging the effectiveness of special education. By its very nature, meta-analysis produces summary statements that are more precise, more dispassionate, and more detached than other review techniques. When, however such conclusions encounter positive intuitive appeal and strong advocacy, it is difficult to dislodge the method in question through evidence and reason. The disagreement involves advocacy and the less-than-disinterested view held by Dunn, who has

a substantial stake in modality-based instruction, assessment devices (Dunn, Dunn, & Price, 1970), and intervention techniques (Dunn & Dunn, 1978). Dunn (1990) provided a Duke's mixture of interpretation that did little to undermine confidence in the primary conclusions: Modality-based instruction is ineffective. Learning is really a matter of substance over style.

# Conclusion

The question of process training presents a vexing situation for special education. For psycholinguistic training, benefits were found in some areas, especially with regard to basic language skill. These benefits found suggest that psycholinguistic training is not an all-or-none proposition, and caution must be exercised lest "the baby get thrown out with the bath water." The cases for perceptual-motor training and modality training appear quite different. In these cases, there were no perceived benefits, and they can be rightly judged in an all-or-none manner with that judgment being unequivocally negative. Yet, they reveal a stubborn resistance to being eliminated from practice. Because of their intuitive appeal and historical foundation and seductive statements found in clinical reports, perceptual-motor training and modality training remain established practices in the special education repertoire of techniques.

The attacks on process training (Mann, 1971b; Mann & Phillips, 1967 ) have been vigorous but apparently not convincing to a segment of special education practitioners. Why? Because processes are presumed to possess a reality that then assumes they must be considered in remedial planning. For a process like language that is reasonably well understood and readily observed, this assumption is probably true and accounts for the selected benefits of psycholinguistic training. These assumptions, however, were not supported for perceptual-motor training and modality training where perception, learning style, and the like are not well understood and certainly not obvious. The empirical evaluation of these methods was decidedly negative but apparently not negative enough to alter fundamental belief. This belief sets in motion an attitude of questioning about research findings typically centered around the notion, "What if . . .?" The tension between belief and reality provides a continuing sense of justification for process training. When historical considerations are also included, process training becomes an entrenched element in special education.

Debate about the efficacy of process training becomes centered on philosophical issues that are not so easily resolved. Regardless of the weight of research evidence against it, process training with its established clinical, historical, and philosophical foundation has proven remarkably resistant as suggested by Mann (1979):

> Process training has always made the phoenix look like a bedraggled sparrow. You cannot kill it. It simply bides its time in exile after being dislodged by one of history's periodic attacks upon it and then returns, wearing disguises or carrying new *noms de plume*, as it were, but consisting of the same old ideas, doing business much in the same old way. (p. 539)

# CHAPTER 4
# RELATED MEDICAL INTERVENTIONS

Just as special education has roots in psychology as demonstrated in the models of learning ability for individuals with MR discussed in chapter 2 and the process training methods primarily for individuals with LD discussed in chapter 3, medicine has long contributed to intervention efforts in special education. Special education practitioners have often turned to medicine, and this has resulted in related medical interventions becoming an integral part of special education. The field of medicine has also shown an interest in schools, and the interface between medicine and special education has made some special education practice medically based. This interface has been evidenced in drug treatment that is often integral to the treatment regimen for individuals with LD and its subsets (e.g., attention deficit/hyperactivity disorder) but also for individuals with MR, where it has also been a source of controversy (see King, State, Davanzo, Shah, & Dykens, 1997; State, King, & Dykens, 1997).

## Stimulant Medication and Hyperactivity

The practice of treating hyperactivity [the preferred terminology is now attention deficit/hyperactivity disorder (ADHD), but the review was completed when hyperactivity was the more common designation] with stimulant drugs is among the most controversial and emotionally loaded issues faced by special education. For some time, the medical community has considered stimulant drugs to be an efficacious treatment for hyperactivity (e.g., American Academy of Pediatrics, 1970, 1975;

Barkley, 1977), and it continues to be used today with about one million students with ADHD being treated with stimulant medication (DuPaul & Stoner, 1994; Safer, 1995). This conclusion, however, has been challenged: first, in the form of critical reviews suggesting no positive interpretation could be drawn from the available research literature because of numerous methodological flaws (e.g., Sprague & Werry, 1971; Sroufe, 1975); and second, in the form of ideological, ethical, and moral attacks upon stimulant drug treatment (e.g., Schrag & Divoky, 1975).

Kavale (1982a) found 135 studies assessing the effectiveness of stimulant medication for the treatment of hyperactivity. The studies sampled represented approximately 5,300 subjects averaging 8.75 years of age with an average IQ of 102; subjects received medication for an average of 10 weeks. The $\overline{ES}$ across 984 *ES* measurements was .58, which indicates that the average treated subject moved from the 50th to the 72nd percentile as a result of drug intervention. This 22-percentile-rank gain suggests that an average subject treated with stimulant medication would be expected to be better off than 72% of untreated control subjects.

The diverse assortment of outcomes measured in drug research makes it difficult to interpret a single index of drug efficacy. Two major outcome classes were identified: behavioral and cognitive. The findings are displayed in Table 17. This more refined analysis revealed substantial positive effects for both behavioral and cognitive outcomes.

# Table 17. Average Effect Size for Stimulant Medication Outcome Assessments

|  | Number of Effect Sizes | Mean Effect Size | Percentile Equivalent |
|---|---|---|---|
| *Behavioral* | | | |
| Global improvement ratings | 192 | .89 | 81 |
| Rating scales and checklists | 113 | .84 | 80 |
| Activity level | 127 | .85 | 80 |
| Attention and concentration | 119 | .78 | 78 |
| Behavior (social and classroom) | 92 | .63 | 74 |
| Anxiety | 12 | .12 | 55 |
| *Cognitive* | | | |
| Intelligence | 54 | .39 | 65 |
| Achievement | 47 | .38 | 65 |
| Drawing and copying | 38 | .47 | 68 |
| Perceptual-motor | 91 | .41 | 66 |
| Learning characteristics | 41 | .37 | 64 |

With the exception of anxiety, impressive gains were found for behavioral outcomes. Substantial benefits were found on ratings of behavioral functioning, lowered activity levels, and improved attending skills. Cognitive functioning also exhibited positive improvement although not of the same magnitude as behavioral improvements. With respect to cognitive tasks, the present findings were generally in accord with findings from laboratory studies regarding the salutary effects of stimulant medication on tasks that tap various aspects of attention and memory (for reviews, see Cantwell & Carlson, 1978; Gittelman & Kanner, 1986). Unlike past reviews (e.g., Aman, 1980; Barkley & Cunningham, 1978), the meta-analytic findings also showed stimulant medication to have a positive effect on academic performance. Students treated with stimulant medication could, in fact, be expected to gain about 15 percentile ranks on achievement measures when compared to nontreated students. To put this achievement gain in perspective, note that meta-analyses have found that interventions deemed just as controversial as psychopharmacological treatment (e.g., perceptual-motor training, modality instruction) have resulted in gains of only 5 or 6 percentile ranks (Forness & Kavale, 1988).

There appears to be resistance, however, to acknowledging any positive effects of medication on academic achievement (e.g., Gadow, 1983; O'Leary, 1980). Any enhanced academic performance is usually attributed to improved attention and reduced impulsivity. When, however, the effects of attention were held constant in the meta-analysis (through partial correlation), the positive effect for achievement was reduced by only 20%, suggesting that factors other than attention were also operating to enhance academic performance.

Pelham (1986) has also questioned the validity of negative conclusions obtained in studies of stimulant medication effects on achievement. It was suggested that the studies suffered from methodological difficulties that limited their findings and included such factors as (a) insensitivity of achievement tests over the typically short (4–12 weeks) duration of medication studies, (b) lack of attention to drug-dose factors, (c) lack of compliance in administering medication, (d) lack of attention to the time course of stimulant effects, and (e) lack of attention to individual differences. Pelham suggested that the presumed positive effects of applied behavior analysis had resulted in an antimedication bias, and different evidential standards were being applied to drug studies. These cautions suggest that negative findings should not necessarily be interpreted as evidence that stimulant medication has no beneficial effect on academic achievement. For example, the $\overline{\text{ES}}$ s for achievement measures from the present meta-analysis are shown in Table 18. With the exception of arithmetic, the gains in academic achievement represent a level of improvement equal to approximately a half-year's worth of schooling ($\overline{\text{ES}} = .50$); the effects of drug treatment exhibit this achievement gain in only 10 weeks.

Drug research has been criticized on methodological grounds, but no significant differences were found among $\overline{\text{ES}}$ s for studies rated as low, medium, or high with respect to internal validity (see Campbell & Stanley, 1966). Design problems thus appeared to play a subordinate role; design considerations accounted for only 1% of the variance in study findings for the behavioral and cognitive classes. Among the more important design elements is placebo control; the comparison group is given an inert substance ("sugar pill"), and if improvement is demonstrated, the gain may be attributed to the placebo effect and doubt cast upon observed drug effects. The difference between placebo controlled studies ($\overline{\text{ES}} = .56$) and studies without placebo control ($\overline{\text{ES}} = .63$) was not significant. The $\overline{\text{ES}}$ difference (.07) can be considered an approximate index of the placebo effect and is well below the standard value (approximately 35%),

## Table 18. Average Effect Size for Stimulant Medication on Achievement Measures

| Measure | Number of Effect Sizes | Mean Effect Size | Percentile Equivalent |
|---|---|---|---|
| Wide Range Achievement Test | | | |
|     Reading | 11 | .32 | 63 |
|     Arithmetic | 10 | .09 | 54 |
|     Spelling | 7 | .37 | 64 |
| Iowa Test of Basic Skills | 6 | .63 | 74 |
| Gray Oral Reading Test | 3 | .42 | 66 |
| Language | 6 | .50 | 69 |
| Handwriting | 4 | .44 | 67 |

which indicates that the placebo effect accounted for only 7% of the improvement shown by drug-treated subjects.

Treatment with stimulant medication appears to be an effective intervention for the treatment of hyperactivity. Compare this conclusion with a statement from a narrative review of the literature: "Our analysis of the literature in this area indicates that research findings do not indicate the general efficacy and therefore do not support the widespread use of stimulant drugs" (Adelman & Compas, 1977, p. 406). The present findings demonstrated that stimulant medication effects produced substantive positive outcomes where the average subject treated with stimulant medication would be better off than 72% of control subjects. No empirical analysis, however, can hope to elucidate the complex ideological and moral issues associated with drug intervention. The controversy over the use of stimulant medication has not abated (e.g., Frankenberger, Lozar, & Dallas, 1990; Wilens & Biederman, 1992), and there is increased concern that stimulant medication may be viewed as a cure (e.g., Combrinck-Graham, 1987; Cowart, 1988). Nevertheless, stimulant medication remains the most prevalent treatment modality for ADHD and has generated a tremendous volume of research (Carlson & Rapport, 1989). Because the Kavale (1982a) meta-analysis is some 15 years old, an updated meta-analytic review is certainly warranted. Additionally, the change in focus from hyperactivity to inattentiveness suggests a shift in the nature of the samples studied, and availability of improved evaluation/ assessment instruments (e.g., Barkley, 1990) suggests that better data are being obtained.

Crenshaw (1997) performed a meta-analysis on the research published between 1981 and 1995, and generally used the same procedures and criteria used by Kavale (1982a) to permit comparison and continuation. The search yielded 115 studies, with 70 including subjects with a diagnosis of ADD; 33, diagnosis of ADHD; 2, both diagnoses; and 10, a generalized diagnosis (e.g., hyperactive). The average age was 9.40 years and average IQ was 99; subjects received medication for an average of 6 weeks. The most often studied psychostimulant was methylphenidate ($n$ = 103). Across 115 studies, the $\overline{ES}$ was .64, which was slightly larger but comparable to the $\overline{ES}$ of .58 found by Kavale. The $\overline{ES}$ of .64 obtained by Crenshaw means that the average drug-treated subject moved from the 50th to the 74th percentile. This is also comparable to Kavale's findings of a 22-percentile-rank increase.

On behavioral outcome measures, Crenshaw (1997) obtained an $\overline{ES}$ of .74, comparable to the behavior $\overline{ES}$ of .80 found by Kavale (1982a). Improved behavior would thus be demonstrated by 74% and 80% of drug-treated subjects in the Crenshaw and Kavale studies respectively when compared to untreated control subjects. With respect to academic outcomes, greater differences between the meta-analyses were found. The Crenshaw study obtained an $\overline{ES}$ of .46 compared to the $\overline{ES}$ of .38 found by Kavale. The positive improvement, however, was similar and amounted to only a 3-percentile-rank difference (68 vs. 65), meaning that the average drug-treated subject demonstrates, on average, a 17-percentile-rank academic outcome gain. The differences between meta-analyses is accounted for primarily by findings for achievement tests (e.g., Wide Range Achievement Test). The Kavale study included almost entirely standardized achievement measures, while the Crenshaw study included more classroom-type assessments (e.g., percentage of work completed). In the Crenshaw analysis, the $\overline{ES}$ for achievement tests was .25 compared to an $\overline{ES}$ of .52 for classroom-type measures. With classroom measures, students on stimulant medication demonstrated academic skills more than one-half *SD* above the average student in the control group.

Thus, in an extension of a meta-analysis published in 1982, Crenshaw (1997) also found positive effects that were quite comparable to the Kavale (1982a) findings. With studies published between 1980 and 1995, similar findings emerged with behavioral outcomes showing a stronger drug response than academic outcomes. Since 1980, with revised diagnostic criteria, more reliable assessment instruments, and more emphasis on behavioral observation, the conclusion attesting to the efficacy of stimulant medication on behavioral and academic outcomes has been affirmed.

# Diet Treatment and Hyperactivity

The influence of medical interventions on special education is exemplified in the case of the "Feingold diet," an intervention for hyperactivity that was popularized during the mid-1970s as a natural alternative to stimulant medication. Although the proliferation of the Feingold Associations (see "Food color link," 1980) promoting the use of the diet to treat hyperactivity has abated, the Feingold diet had significant impact on special education. Dr. Benjamin Feingold (1975) offered the hypothesis that the ingestion of artificial (synthetic) food additives (colors and flavors) contributes to hyperactivity (Feingold, 1976). The

suggested treatment was based upon the tenets of the Feingold Kaiser-Permanente (K-P) diet designed to eliminate all foods containing any artificial food additives from the diet (Feingold & Feingold, 1979).

Feingold (1976) reported that from 40% to 70% of subjects demonstrated a marked reduction in hyperactive behavior as a result of diet modification. The available evidence, based upon uncontrolled clinical trials and anecdotal accounts, was challenged but, nevertheless, the Feingold K-P diet received widespread media attention as well as a favorable and enthusiastic response from the general public. The question thus remained: Is there any justification for the major dietary changes required by the Feingold K-P diet in terms of reduced hyperactivity?

Kavale and Forness (1983) examined 23 experimental studies assessing the efficacy of the Feingold K-P diet in treating hyperactivity. The 23 studies produced 125 *ES* measurements, and yielded an $\overline{ES}$ of .12 but a median *ES* of .05, suggesting a skewed distribution with the $\overline{ES}$ probably overestimating the treatment effect. The average subject was 8.3 years of age, had an IQ of 99, and remained on the Feingold K-P diet for 39 weeks.

In relative terms, the $\overline{ES}$ of .12 indicates that a subject no better off than average (i.e., at the 50th percentile) would rise to the 55th percentile as a result of the Feingold K-P diet. When compared to the 22-percentile-rank gain for treatment with stimulant medication, the 5-percentile-rank improvement for diet modification is less than one-fourth as large. Although the average ages and IQ were similar for drug-treated and diet-treated subjects, the average duration of treatment differed: 39 weeks in a diet

## Table 19. Average Effect Size for Feingold Kaiser-Permanente Diet on Outcome Assessments

| Category | Number of Effect Sizes | Mean Effect Size | Percentile Equivalent |
|---|---|---|---|
| Conners Scale–Parents | 26 | .16 | 56 |
| Conners Scale–Teachers | 9 | .27 | 61 |
| Global improvement rating | 23 | .13 | 55 |
| Hyperkinesis rating | 15 | .29 | 61 |
| Attention | 36 | .02 | 51 |
| Disruptive behavior | 6 | .05 | 52 |
| Impulsivity | 5 | .15 | 56 |
| Learning ability | 10 | −.06 | 48 |

study and 10 weeks in a drug study. In relation to $\overline{ES}$ (.12 vs. .58), these comparisons suggest that compared to Feingold K-P diet treatment, treatment with stimulant medication is approximately five times as effective in about one-fourth the time. Thus, the Feingold K-P diet is cast in an unfavorable light since it produces a substantially lower treatment effect than stimulant medication while approximating the negligible effects of, for example, perceptual-motor training ($\overline{ES}$ = .08).

The ES data were next aggregated into descriptive outcome categories, and the findings are shown in Table 19. The effects of the Feingold K-P diet ranged from a loss of 2 percentile ranks (learning ability) to gains of 11 percentile ranks (Conners Scale–Teachers and hyperkinesis ratings). Thus, the only obvious effect of treatment through diet modification is upon overt behavior, specifically a perceived reduction in hyperactivity. This conclusion, however, must be tempered; global ratings of improvement possess two major problems: objectivity in defining improvement and psychometric deficiencies (reliability and validity).

These problems influence the "reactivity" or subjectivity of outcome measures; the measures are under the control of observers who have an acknowledged interest in achieving predetermined outcomes (e.g., "improvement"). Nonreactive measures, on the other hand, are not easily influenced in any direction by observers. The correlation of ES and ratings of reactivity ($r$ = .18) was significant, suggesting that larger treatment effects were associated with more reactive measures. Additionally, aggregations of reactive versus nonreactive measures found $\overline{ES}$s of .18 and .01 respectively, suggesting that in those instances where instruments paralleled the valued outcomes of observers, there was tendency to view greater improvement.

The initial evaluations of diet modification by Dr. Feingold and associates were based upon clinical trial and observation. Such findings, however, are at variance with findings from "better" studies, that is, those studies that included more rigorous experimental control. Of the 23 studies, the 6 uncontrolled clinical trials yielded an $\overline{ES}$ of .34

compared to the $\overline{ES}$ of .09 for the 17 controlled studies. There was, however, a significant relationship ($r = -.19$) between $ES$ and ratings of design quality, indicating that larger $ES$s were associated with studies rated low on internal validity.

The 17 controlled studies used two primary experimental designs. The first was a diet crossover study that placed groups of subjects on two experimental diets: One group followed the Feingold K-P diet strictly, while the other was disguised as the Feingold K-P diet but actually contained the substances supposedly eliminated. The second design was a challenge study, in which subjects who appeared to respond to the Feingold K-P diet were selected and divided into experimental and control groups. Both groups were placed on a strict Feingold K-P diet, and at the end of the trial the experimental group was "challenged" with a food (usually a cookie or drink) that contained large doses of the eliminated substances.

Of the 17 controlled studies, 7 used a diet crossover design and 10 were challenge studies. The diet crossover studies yielded an $\overline{ES}$ of .20, and the challenge studies produced an $\overline{ES}$ of .05. Challenge studies offer a design that permits the attribution of behavioral change to the substances eliminated in the Feingold K-P diet; they can be considered the "best" studies and provide the most convincing evidence for evaluating the efficacy of the Feingold K-P diet. The weight of this evidence, however, is decidedly negative ($\overline{ES} = .05$); at the end of diet modification, the average treatment subject was at the 52nd percentile compared to the 50th percentile of control subjects, a gain only slightly better than no treatment at all.

These meta-analytic findings offer little support for the Feingold hypothesis. The modest and limited gains found suggest a more temperate view of the efficacy of the Feingold K-P diet than that asserted by the diet's proponents. The negative evaluation of the Feingold diet has found support in previous reviews (e.g., Mattes, 1983; National Advisory Committee on Hyperkinesis and Food Additives, 1980; Stare, Whelan, & Sheridan, 1980), but has appeared to have little effect on the steadfastness of belief about the efficacy of the Feingold diet. Instead, attention was directed at a number of possible defects in the available research studies. For example, Rimland (1983) discussed six supposed defects in the available studies that presumably make them irrelevant, and concluded with the warning, "What is the cost to us, to our country, and to our civilization of allowing ourselves to be seduced into consuming the gaudy colors and deceptive flavors that are used to make non-nutritious food appear desirable?" (p. 333). Setting aside this hyperbole, the empirical evidence appears sound and suggests that artificial additives serve merely a cosmetic function with no negative effects on behavior and learning (see Mattes, 1983). The use of the Feingold diet appears to be predicated not on research evidence, which is decidedly negative, but rather on sociological factors like the desire for a natural treatment and a distrust of food manufacturers. These are not sufficient grounds for dismissing more critical empirical evaluations of the Feingold K-P diet because more appropriate medical, psychological, or educational intervention may be postponed (Conners, 1980; Wender, 1977).

Although the Feingold K-P diet offers an appealing treatment approach for hyperactivity by offering a natural alternative to stimulant medication, it is not without pragmatic difficulties. The implementation of the Feingold K-P diet requires an abrupt lifestyle change. Increased vigilance is necessary, for example, in grocery shopping and food preparation, families generally cannot eat at restaurants, and the student cannot eat school lunches (Sheridan & Meister, 1982). Lew (1977) conducted a 4-week trial of the Feingold K-P diet and concluded that "the Feingold Diet is indeed a very different and very difficult diet to maintain in practice. The deprivations to the participants are real and is not the hyperactive child already set apart from his peers and family enough?" (p. 190). The negative findings from the meta-analysis call into question the validity of the Feingold K-P diet as a treatment for hyperactivity and suggest a cautious policy toward accepting the Feingold hypothesis.

# Psychotropic Medication

The 1950s marked the beginning of a new treatment approach for severe behavior disorders: psychotropic medication. With severe behavior disorders an integral part of the special education "serious emotional disturbance" category, treatment with psychotropic medication became a significant adjunct therapy associated with special education. Much like the case of stimulant medication in the treatment of ADHD, however, psychotropic medication for the treatment of serious emotional disturbance has provoked controversy. Early reports (e.g., Campbell, 1975a, 1975b; Fish, 1960) suggested salutary effects, but later evaluations (e.g., Klein, Gittelman, Quitkin, & Riffkin, 1980; Werry, 1982) suggested more caution because, while positive effects were

present, they were not sufficient to affect the most important clinical features associated with severe behavior disorders. With mixed findings about efficacy, it has been difficult to provide answers to the questions: What are the overall therapeutic benefits of psychotropic medication on severe behavior disorders? On what kinds of outcome measures has drug treatment had the greatest effects? Which individuals have benefited most from treatment with psychotropic medication?

Kavale and Nye (1984) reviewed 70 studies examining the effects of psychotropic medication in the treatment of severe behavior disorders. A total of about 4,000 subjects were represented who averaged 16.25 years of age with an average IQ of 84; the average treatment period was 9 weeks. Across 401 $ES$ measurements, the $\overline{ES}$ was .30, which indicates that the average subject receiving psychotropic medication moved from the 50th to the 62nd percentile; the average subject was thus better off than 62% of subjects not treated with psychotropic medication. Of 401 $ES$ measurements, 33% were negative, indicating a 67% positive response to drug treatment.

With respect to behavioral and cognitive outcomes, $\overline{ES}$s of .28 and .74 were found, respectively. When compared to subjects not receiving psychotropic medication, the gains for drug-treated subjects translate into 9- and 27-percentile-rank increases for behavioral and cognitive outcomes respectively. The specific categories associated with behavioral and cognitive outcomes are displayed in Table 20.

The largest $\overline{ES}$ in the behavioral category was found for improvement ratings that included both global assessments and standardized scales. Although criticized for problems related to objectivity and problematic psychometric properties (see Conners, 1973), behavior ratings have been found sensitive to improved behavioral functioning, and the 19-percentile-rank gain for subjects treated with psychotropic medication cannot be easily discounted (Conners & Werry, 1979). The self-help category revealed an increase amounting to 15 percentile ranks and, because the measures assess overt behaviors (e.g., dressing, eating, toileting) that are more directly and objectively measured, the positive findings are likely an accurate reflection of positive effects for medication. The remaining outcome categories (socialization and school behavior) exhibited little or no change. For subjects treated with psychotropic medication, school behavior improved a modest 6 percentile ranks, while 2 percentile ranks were lost on measures of social skill.

Measures of cognitive skill found drug-treated subjects better off than 71% of subjects not receiving psychotropic medication. The 17-percentile-rank gain on measures of attention and concentration suggests an approximate 70% reduction in error scores on tasks assessing these processes. The greatest gain was found on measures of intellectual performance, where the $\overline{ES}$ (.97) amounts to an IQ increase of about 14 points for the average subject receiving psychotropic medication. It is not possible, however, to determine how direct or indirect are the effects related to intelligence. For example, do the IQ gains represent only improved functioning resulting from enhanced attention? The remaining cognitive categories revealed positive gains, but the small number of *ESs* limits interpretation.

Three major drug types were used most frequently: stimulants, major

## Table 20. Average Effect Size for Psychotropic Medication on Behavior and Cognitive Outcome Assessments

| Outcome Category | Number of Effect Sizes | Mean Effect Size | Percentile Equivalent |
|---|---|---|---|
| *Behavior* | | | |
| Improvement ratings | 157 | .49 | 69 |
| Self-help | 14 | .39 | 65 |
| Socialization | 144 | −.05 | 48 |
| School behavior | 10 | .16 | 56 |
| *Cognitive* | | | |
| Attention/Concentration | 25 | .46 | 67 |
| Intelligence | 23 | .97 | 83 |
| Achievement | 3 | .11 | 54 |
| Paired-associate learning | 4 | .76 | 78 |
| Verbalization | 6 | .38 | 65 |
| Perception | 3 | .33 | 63 |

tranquilizers, and antidepressants. The findings for each drug group are shown in Table 21. Although major tranquilizers appear to be the drug of choice, the $\overline{ES}$ difference between tranquilizers and stimulants was negligible, and both approximate the overall effect ($\overline{ES} = .30$). The gain associated with antidepressants is impressive, but must be approached with caution because of the small number of *ESs*.

The effects by diagnostic category are shown in Table 22. The largest $\overline{ES}$ was found for "severe emotional disturbance," composed of subjects with specific diagnoses (e.g., schizophrenia, autism, atypical development), while the smallest $\overline{ES}$ was found for "severe behavior disturbance," defined by subjects with undifferentiated psychosis diagnoses. Although largely undifferentiated, organically based severe behavior

disorders revealed a larger $\overline{ES}$ than undifferentiated nonorganic psychotic disorders. A significant correlation between *ES* and specificity of diagnosis indicates more impressive drug effects associated with more specific diagnostic classifications.

Table 23 shows effects for different age groupings. The largest $\overline{ES}$ was found for the young adult grouping, with the remaining groupings falling below the overall $\overline{ES}$ (.30). A significant difference was found between young adults and adolescents. There was also a significant correlation between *ES* and age, which indicates a trend for larger *ES* being associated with older subjects. Psychotropic medication appears most beneficial for the age range 16 to 25 years, where drug-treated subjects are better off than 96% of non-drug-treated young adults.

## Table 21. Average Effect Size for Psychotropic Medication

| Medication Type | Number of Effect Sizes | Mean Effect Size | Percentile Equivalent |
|---|---|---|---|
| Stimulant | 97 | .25 | 60 |
| Tranquilizer (antipsychotic) | 288 | .28 | 61 |
| Antidepressant | 4 | 1.22 | 89 |

## Table 22. Average Effect Size for Psychotropic Medication by Diagnostic Category

| Diagnostic Category | Number of Effect Sizes | Mean Effect Size | Percentile Equivalent |
|---|---|---|---|
| Severe emotional disturbance (specific psychosis classification) | 83 | .57 | 72 |
| Severe behavior disturbance (undifferentiated psychosis classification) | 211 | .11 | 54 |
| Organically based severe behavior disorder | 101 | .43 | 67 |

## Table 23.  Average Effect Size
## for Psychotropic Medication by Age Group

| Age Group | Number of Effect Sizes | Mean Effect Size | Percentile Equivalent |
|---|---|---|---|
| Child (1–8 years) | 42 | .21 | 58 |
| Adolescent (9–15 years) | 207 | .13 | 55 |
| Young Adult (16–25 years) | 12 | 1.74 | 96 |
| Adult (26+ years) | 15 | .26 | 60 |

The findings suggest the presence of therapeutic benefits from psychotropic medication in the treatment of severe behavior disorders. In general, psychotropic medication was found to produce consistent, albeit modest, positive effects. When compared to other drug therapies, the effects of psychotropic medication on severe behavior disorders (.30) were not of the magnitude found for either hyperactivity ($\overline{ES}$ = .58; see Kavale, 1982a) or adult psychological disturbance ($\overline{ES}$ = .51; see Smith, Glass, & Miller, 1980). In these meta-analyses approximately 72% of students with hyperactivity and 70% of adult psychological patients would be better off than untreated control subjects, compared to the 62% improvement found here for subjects with severe behavior disorders. The most likely explanation for the approximate 10-percentile-rank advantage found in the other meta-analyses is severity level; for example, only one-third of the adult patients were psychotic. More severe behavior disorders cannot be expected to improve as much as milder forms of behavior disorder as a result of drug intervention. Nevertheless, the findings related to psychotropic medication suggest it to be an important component in the management of severe behavior disorders. Given the date (1984) of the Kavale and Nye meta-analysis, an updated meta-analysis like the Crenshaw study for stimulant medication is certainly warranted to permit comparison and continuation in the investigation of the efficacy of psychotropic medication.

## Conclusion

The meta-analytic findings about medically based interventions suggest that they are a useful part of special education. In comparison to interventions emanating from special education, medically based interventions appear no better or worse. The case of hyperactivity (or ADHD) demonstrates why this is the case: One form (stimulant medication) was effective while the other (diet modification) was not. For severe behavior disorders, drug treatment produced modest positive effects, suggesting that psychotropic medication is best viewed as only part of a total treatment program. The findings suggest that special education should temper any particular fascination with medically based interventions. They require the same critical evaluation as other forms of interventions and, as demonstrated, may be judged as more or less appropriate for inclusion in a special education program.

# CHAPTER 5
# SOCIAL SKILLS TRAINING

A relatively new intervention that has received considerable attention is social skills training. Efficacy in social relationships is not only a primary goal of parents or caretakers for children with MR or other disabilities (Westling, 1996), but is also integral to the notion of empowerment for all individuals with disabilities (Polloway et al., 1996). The goal of social skills training is thus to enhance the social functioning of special education students. Walker, Colvin, and Ramsey (1995) have defined social skills as a set of competencies that allows students to initiate and maintain positive social relationships with others, to establish positive peer acceptance and satisfactory school adjustment, and to cope effectively and adaptively with the larger social environment. Social skills training typically includes such components as teaching the identification of prosocial behaviors and strategies, modeling such behaviors and strategies, practicing these prosocial skills in simulated or real-life settings, and teaching students to self-monitor, self-evaluate, and self-reinforce skills in various situations (Rutherford, Chipman, DiGangi, & Anderson, 1992).

Although it is not clear how social skill deficits develop (e.g., Gresham, 1992), efforts directed at enhancing these skills have been undertaken, but evaluations of the efforts have produced mixed findings regarding efficacy (e.g., Gresham, 1981; McIntosh, Vaughn, & Zaragoza, 1991; Zaragoza, Vaughn, & McIntosh, 1991). The difficulties in reaching firm conclusions about the effectiveness of social skills training are partially related to problems in delineat-ing what actually constitutes social skills training (e.g., Pray, Hall, & Markley, 1992). as well as difficulties in establishing a link between identified social skill deficits and specific components of training (e.g., Gresham, 1986; Strain, Guralnik, & Walker, 1986). Similarly, training components are not always well-described, outcome variables are not consistently measured by psychometrically sound instruments (Maag, 1989), and contextual variables that may contribute to adverse social interactions are frequently not acknowledged (Gresham, 1993; Maag, 1993).

## Social Skills Training for Students With Learning Disabilities

Beginning in the 1970s, there was increasing recognition that students with LD not only manifested academic difficulties, but were also at risk for problems in the social domain. Social skill deficits are now recognized as part of the LD symptom complex (Bryan, 1991; LaGreca & Vaughn, 1992; Pearl, 1992); the deficits range from general problems in social cognition (Pearl, 1987) and social behavior (LaGreca, 1987) to more specific deficits related to peer status (Dudley-Marling & Edmiaston, 1985) and self-concept (Chapman, 1988). The recognition of social deficits among students with LD led to efforts to ameliorate those deficits, and a number of different training programs have been developed for that purpose (Kavale & Forness, 1995). Their efficacy, however, remains open to question (e.g., Schumaker & Hazel, 1988; Swanson & Malone, 1992;

Vaughn, 1991), and much of the tentativeness about the effectiveness of social skills training is due partially to problems with the research literature that limit its interpretation (Asher & Taylor, 1983; Ladd, 1984).

Forness and Kavale (1996b) synthesized data from 52 studies investigating the effectiveness of social skills training for students with LD. The studies included 2,113 subjects who averaged 11.5 years of age with an average IQ of 96; subjects received training for approximately 3 hours per week across 10 weeks. The 52 studies produced 328 $ES$ measurements with an $\overline{ES}$ of .21; the median $ES$ was .18, suggesting a positive skew. Of the 328 $ES$ measures, 22% were negative, suggesting that in about 1 in 5 instances social skills training actually produced better gains in the control (untrained) rather than the experimental (trained) group.

In relative terms, the $\overline{ES}$ of .21 suggests that an average student with LD (i.e., at the 50th percentile) would only rise to the 58th percentile as a result of social skills training, indicating only

modest gains. Using Cohen's (1988) classification of $ES$ magnitude, the $\overline{ES}$ of .21 would be termed small. There were, however, differences in the way that teachers, peers, and students themselves evaluated the outcome of social skills training.

When students with LD evaluated themselves on outcomes, the largest $\overline{ES}$ for training was obtained. These findings could be aggregated across six dimensions and are shown in Table 24. The $\overline{ES}$ across 117 measures in which self-report or self-rating by students with LD were obtained was .24, an effect that would leave the average student with LD better off than 59% of students receiving no social skills training. The largest $\overline{ES}$ was found for social status, where 65% of students with LD perceived an improved status. Apparently, students with LD, after receiving training, believed that their social status was enhanced, while their peers without LD who assessed the effects of the same training perceived no such improvement. Better than 6 out of 10 students with LD also perceived benefits from social skills training in the areas of

## Table 24. Average Effect Size for Self-Assessments of Social Skills Training for Students With Learning Disabilities

| Components | Number of Effect Sizes | Mean Effect Size | Percentile Equivalent |
|---|---|---|---|
| Social status | 16 | .38 | 65 |
| Self-concept | 24 | .28 | 61 |
| Social problem solving | 11 | .28 | 61 |
| Social competence | 30 | .27 | 61 |
| Interaction | 17 | .19 | 58 |
| Locus of control | 19 | .08 | 53 |
| Self-assessment composite mean | 117 | .24 | 59 |

## Table 25. Average Effect Size for General Education Peer Assessments of Social Skills Training for Students With Learning Disabilities

| Components | Number of Effect Sizes | Mean Effect Size | Percentile Equivalent |
|---|---|---|---|
| Communication | 19 | .25 | 60 |
| Acceptance | 25 | .23 | 59 |
| Cooperation | 13 | .22 | 59 |
| Friendship | 13 | .22 | 59 |
| Rejection | 23 | .20 | 58 |
| Interaction | 24 | .20 | 58 |
| Social status | 21 | .13 | 55 |
| Peer assessment composite mean | 138 | .21 | 58 |

self-concept, social problem solving, and social competence, but fewer perceived improvement in social interactions or locus of control.

General education peers evaluated the effects of social skills training for their classmates with LD somewhat more modestly. The $\overline{ES}$ across seven dimensions was .21, as shown in Table 25. Peers found the greatest advantage for social skills training in the area of communicative competence; about 60% of students with LD were seen by classmates as improved in their ability to understand the dynamics of communication in social settings. Social status of their classmates was perceived to be the least improved area, while five other areas concerned with social integration clustered around the $\overline{ES}$ (.21). The overall level of improvement was only slightly above chance, and suggests that general education peers were somewhat more amenable to integrating students with LD but did not change the view that their counterparts retained an inferior status.

Teachers' evaluations of social skills training could be aggregated across six dimensions and are the least sanguine; the findings are shown in Table 26. The $\overline{ES}$ across 73 measures was .16. About 6 out of 10 students with LD were perceived by teachers to be slightly better adjusted and less dependent as the result of social interventions. Conduct disorder was seen as slightly more improved, while hyperactivity (i.e., non-goal-directed behavior) was essentially unimproved, at least in the perception of teachers. Teachers also perceived little improvement in academic competence and social interaction.

Differences in $\overline{ES}$ among the three groups assessing outcomes were not significant. Although the largest effect of social skills training was found in the evaluations performed by students with LD themselves, the $\overline{ES}$ translated only into a modest 9-percentile-rank gain. Regardless of who did the evaluation, however, it appears that such training resulted in relatively minimal gains.

## Table 26. Average Effect Size for Teacher Assessments of Social Skills Training for Students With Learning Disabilities

| Training Program | Number of Effect Sizes | Mean Effect Size | Percentile Equivalent |
|---|---|---|---|
| Adjustment | 15 | .29 | 62 |
| Dependency | 10 | .25 | 60 |
| Conduct disorder | 8 | .22 | 59 |
| Interaction | 17 | .11 | 54 |
| Hyperactivity | 9 | .07 | 53 |
| Academic competence | 14 | .05 | 52 |
| Teacher assessment composite mean | 73 | .16 | 56 |

Although social skills deficits are among the primary characteristics of students with LD, these deficits appear resistant to treatment. Across more than 50 studies, training effects were modest; in better than 1 in 5 studies, control groups actually showed more improvement than experimental groups. There were some differences among teachers, peers, and students with LD themselves in their perceptions about the beneficial effects, but these differences proved to be insignificant.

Among evaluators, students with LD themselves were the most impressed with their social skills after training. However, general education peers tended to view the same findings as significantly less positive. Although students with LD ranked their social status as the most improved area, their general education peers rated social status as the least improved area. Teacher impressions were quite modest regarding the impact of training on overall social adjustment, and almost negligible regarding the benefits of intervention for such problems as conduct disorders and hyperactivity.

Teachers rated academic competence as virtually unaffected by such training. All three groups rated actual social interaction among the least improved skills.

Why did such a widely used intervention prove to be such a disappointment? A number of possibilities exist. The most obvious involves intensity of training; average time allocated for social skills training tended to be 30 hours or less (i.e., fewer than 3 hours per week for less than 10 weeks). Although length of training was not a significant correlate, the possibility exists that longer interventions might be needed to produce more positive results. Since the average treated student with LD was in the 6th grade, it is not unreasonable to assume that social skill deficits were relatively long-standing; it should then come as no surprise that 30 hours might prove insufficient to ameliorate social problems. Even for intensive interventions over a period of years, there may be only modest outcomes with some students, or some students may respond during some periods and not others (Vaughn & Hogan, 1994).

A second possibility surrounds measurement issues. A number of criticisms have been directed at assessments for social skills (e.g., Forness & Kavale, 1991; Hughes & Sullivan, 1988; Vaughn & Haager, 1994). Examples include poor rationale for selection of items, dubious psychometric properties of instruments, failure to account for contextual or social validity variables that influence expression of social skills, and lack of differentiation between skill and performance deficits. These shortcomings become even more problematic when instruments are used to assess social skill training effects over time. Many studies used in the meta-analysis did not employ recently developed social skills rating scales designed specifically to address these measurement issues (e.g., Gresham & Elliott, 1990; Walker & McConnell, 1988). Careful review of studies also revealed either a vagueness in conception or a lack of concordance between dimensions of social skills being assessed and those being trained (Zaragoza, Vaughn, & McIntosh, 1991). It was thus not always clear that, if an intervention was successful, the outcomes could be demonstrated given available dependent measures.

Training packages themselves represented a third possible reason for lack of significant positive training effects. Almost all studies used a social skills training program specifically designed for research purposes. Such programs usually represented an amalgam of available techniques with no clear rationale and little pilot testing beforehand. There are indeed a number of potentially effective social skills training packages (e.g., Campbell & Siperstein, 1994; Elliott & Gresham, 1991; Hazel, Schumaker, Sherman, & Sheldon-

Wildgen, 1981; McGinnis, Goldstein, Sprafkin, & Gershaw, 1984; Vaughn, Levine, & Ridley, 1986; Walker et al., 1978; Walker et al., 1983), but these were not often used in the studies synthesized. It may well be that social skills training is efficacious, but this fact could not be demonstrated given the intervention programs used nor could effective components be isolated.

A fourth explanation for the disappointing results of social skills training involves controversies surrounding the genesis of social skill deficits in students with LD. If, as one hypothesis suggests, low achievement leads to poor self-esteem or peer rejection, then intervention efforts might be better directed at the primary feature of LD—academic deficits—and not at social skills deficits. If, on the other hand, social skill deficits themselves lead to withdrawal from academic settings or poor self-concept in learning situations, and thus to LD, then social skills training is warranted. This, however, is the least tenuous hypothesis about the link between LD and social competence. If both are presumed to emanate from a common neurologic origin, perhaps the social skills training programs used for students with LD do not possess sufficient emphasis on cognitive, linguistic, or other components that comprise the core of this common etiology.

The possibility cannot be entirely dismissed, however, that the $\overline{ES}$ is a valid indicator of effectiveness for social skills training (i.e., it is a weak intervention or at least one that receives limited empirical support). Social skill deficits continue to characterize students with LD into adulthood and seem to be even more devastating than lack of academic skills in producing poor adult outcomes (Vogel

& Forness, 1992). Beyond the school years, situations requiring social competence tend to far outnumber those requiring academic skill. Competent social presentation may in turn serve to minimize the impact of academic skill deficits. That social skills training has only limited empirical support is discouraging. It is premature, however, to abandon this treatment modality in the absence of further research that might clarify critical factors related to treatment intensity, delineation of training, structure of training programs, and other methodological issues that seem as yet unresolved.

# Social Skills Training for Students With Emotional or Behavioral Disorders

Implicit if not inherent in the definition of E/BD is the concept of deficits in social functioning (Forness & Knitzer, 1992; Kavale & Forness, 1996). Such deficits have naturally led to the development of social skills training programs designed to teach specific interpersonal skills. Social skills training has been used with a wide variety of E/BD from attention deficit disorder (Guevremont & Dumas, 1994) to depression (Asarnow, 1992), and from autism (Kennedy & Shukla, 1995) to delinquency or conduct disorder (Conduct Problems Prevention Research Group, 1992).

Evaluations assessing the effectiveness of social skills training for students with E/BD have generally reached equivocal conclusions (e.g., Hughes & Sullivan, 1988; Mathur & Rutherford, 1991, 1994; Schneider & Byrne, 1985). The equivocation may result partially from sampling problems; few studies investigating social skills training focused

directly on "clinical" samples of students with E/BD (i.e., students identified for special education, mental health, juvenile justice, or related services). A majority of studies used subjects identified primarily by their social skill deficits; but in relatively few instances did studies include subjects identified secondarily, if at all, by their status as possessing E/BD. It cannot be assumed that a subject who has a social skill deficit automatically possesses E/BD, or vice versa.

Kavale, Mathur, Forness, Rutherford, and Quinn (1997) synthesized data from 35 studies investigating the efficacy of social skills training. The studies included 1,123 subjects who averaged 11.5 years of age with an average IQ of 94; subjects received training for about 2 $^1/_2$ hours per week across 12 weeks. The 35 studies produced 328 $ES$ measurements with an $\overline{ES}$ of .20; the median $ES$ was .16, suggesting a modest positive skew. Of 328 $ES$ measurements, 27% were negative, suggesting that in better than 1 in 4 cases, subjects receiving no social skills training achieved better results.

In relative terms, the $\overline{ES}$ of .20 indicates that an average student with E/BD (i.e., at the 50th percentile) would advance to the 58th percentile as a result of social skills training. The 8-percentile-rank gain is modest and, using Cohen's (1988) classification of $ES$ magnitude, would be termed "small." As was the case with social skills training for students with LD, differences were found in the way individuals perceived outcome effectiveness, and the findings for five groups are shown in Table 27.

Teachers perceived the greatest benefit from social skills training, as evidenced by the $\overline{ES}$ of .22. In contrast, parents perceived only limited benefit from social skills training. The difference

## Table 27. Average Effect Size of Social Skills Training by Teacher, Peer, Self, Experimenter, and Parent Assessments of Students With Emotional/Behavioral Disorders

| Rater | Number of Effect Sizes | Mean Effect Size | Percentile Equivalent |
|---|---|---|---|
| Teacher | 73 | .22 | 59 |
| Peer | 44 | .22 | 59 |
| Self | 83 | .22 | 59 |
| Experimenter | 60 | .19 | 58 |
| Parent | 68 | .15 | 56 |
| Rater composite mean | 328 | .20 | 58 |

## Table 28. Average Effect Size of Training on Social Skill Dimensions for Students With Emotional/Behavioral Disorders

| Dimension | Number of Effect Sizes | Mean Effect Size | Percentile Equivalent |
|---|---|---|---|
| Social behavior | 16 | .27 | 61 |
| Social relations | 13 | .27 | 61 |
| Social problem solving | 22 | .26 | 60 |
| Social competence | 21 | .22 | 59 |

was only 3 percentile ranks but demonstrates that adults with the most direct contact with students had different perceptions about outcomes. Students with E/BD and their peers revealed similar perceptions about the effectiveness of social skills training. In both instances, the evaluations were above the overall average level (.20) and showed a gain equivalent to that perceived by teachers (9 percentile ranks). These findings suggest that while social skills training evaluated within a school context was perceived to be effective, this perceived effectiveness apparently did not transfer to the home environment. When

evaluated by experimenters, the $\overline{ES}$ (.19) is below the overall average (.20), but is only 1 percentile rank lower than the largest percentile-rank gain (9). These findings suggest limited variability among raters; and, regardless of who did the rating, social skills training resulted in only modest perceived improvements in social functioning.

The evaluation of social skills training encompasses a number of factors that range from general to specific indices. It is therefore convenient to aggregate ES data into groupings that demonstrate increasing differentiation. Table 28 displays an analysis of the effects of social skills training on broadly defined dimensions.

The dimensions related to social problem solving and social competence were most often evaluated with formal assessments (e.g., Means-End Problem Solving, Test of Social Intelligence, Test of Social Inference), while social behavior and relations were usually evaluated through observational techniques and the perceptions of others. Performance related to these dimensions was enhanced by about 9 to 11 percentile ranks, but the large variability evidenced in the standard deviations associated with social problem solving and social relations suggests caution in interpretation. It

appears that at a general level encompassing broadly based concepts of competence, behavior, and relations in the social realm, training results in moderate improvement; however, the gains were modest and, on average, the student with E/BD receiving social skills training would be better off than only 60% of students not receiving the training.

Four broadly defined areas related to social skills were also identified, and the findings are shown in Table 29. On average, students with E/BD gained about 7 percentile ranks in these social skill areas. Although parents revealed the smallest $\overline{ES}$ (.15) among raters, there was a slightly higher positive effect within the

**Table 29. Average Effect Size of Training on Social Skill Areas for Students With Emotional/Behavioral Disorders**

| Area | Number of Effect Sizes | Mean Effect Size | Percentile Equivalent |
|---|---|---|---|
| Family relations | 9 | .20 | 58 |
| Communication | 28 | .18 | 57 |
| School behavior | 21 | .18 | 57 |
| Conduct disorder | 21 | .13 | 55 |

**Table 30. Average Effect Size of Training on Social Skill Variables for Students With Emotional/Behavioral Disorders**

| Variable | Number of Effect Sizes | Mean Effect Size | Percentile Equivalent |
|---|---|---|---|
| Anxiety | 8 | .42 | 66 |
| Adjustment | 10 | .27 | 61 |
| Cooperation | 12 | .26 | 60 |
| Interaction | 34 | .24 | 59 |
| Self-concept/esteem | 17 | .16 | 56 |
| Aggression | 20 | .13 | 55 |

general area of family relations, suggesting a somewhat more broadly based effect. Communication interaction was enhanced slightly by training, but the $\overline{ES}$ is marked by variability four times greater than the effect, making interpretation problematic.

Social skills training appears to have only limited effect on the symptoms of conduct disorder. The very modest gain (5 percentile ranks) represents almost no improvement and suggests that conduct disorder may be resistant to change. Similarly, although school behavior reveals a slightly larger $\overline{ES}$, it appears that broadly defined aspects of school behavior show limited improvement even though teachers perceived the greatest gain ($\overline{ES} = .22$) among students with E/BD.

On average, the 7-percentile-rank gain demonstrated for social skill areas was modest; the average student with E/BD would be better off than only 57% of students not receiving social skills training.

The findings for six specific outcome variables are displayed in Table 30. The largest obtained $\overline{ES}$ was for anxiety, and it appears that social skills training reduces stress. This positive effect is difficult to interpret, however, in terms of the behavioral functioning of students with E/BD. In contrast, it appears that social skills training has limited influence on improving self-concept/esteem (e.g., Piers-Harris Self-Concept Scale, Coopersmith Self-Esteem Inventory). Thus, it appears that, while students with E/BD experience less anxiety after training, they are not feeling better about themselves, and any positive evaluations are related to factors other than self-concept/esteem.

The variables related to interaction, cooperation, and adjustment clustered together and, on average, the variables defining the ability to relate with others increased by 10 percentile ranks, with the average student with E/BD being better off than 60% of students not receiving social skills training. The positive evaluations noted for teachers, peers, and students with E/BD themselves appeared to be related to the effects found for interaction, cooperation, and adjustment since they represent obvious prosocial behaviors.

A very modest effect was found for aggression. The average student with E/BD demonstrated only a 5-percentile-rank gain that translates into negligible improvement. Since aggression constitutes a primary symptom of conduct disorder, this finding was in accord with the evaluation showing only modest improvement in the area of conduct disorder. It appears that although some aspects of social skill demonstrate modest improvement, aggression and the larger context of conduct disorder were not amenable to training and revealed a resistance to positive change.

With social skill deficits being a primary variable defining students with E/BD, efforts have been directed at ameliorating those deficits through training. The present findings suggest that such efforts met with only limited success; only about 58% of students with E/BD would accrue benefits from social skills training, and the gain would be a modest 8 percentile ranks on an outcome assessment. Across different evaluators, there was limited variation, suggesting that the outcomes of social skills training were perceived similarly, all fell near the 58th percentile equivalent found overall.

The effects of training were evaluated across a variety of social skills, and no substantive differences were found; it was evident that social skills training resulted in only modest improvement for students with E/BD. Regardless of whether the assessed outcome was a broad dimension (e.g., social competence), a more narrowly focused area (e.g., communication), or a specific variable (e.g., aggression), findings consistently revealed training to be of limited value in enhancing social skills.

Analysis of the findings suggests somewhat greater success when the outcomes are focused on social skill factors themselves. Somewhat larger effects, for example, were noted for social problem solving, interaction, cooperation, and assessments based on sociometric procedures that all fall under the rubric of social skills. Conversely, there were smaller effects when the outcomes were part of a larger behavioral realm. For example, social skills training had little effect on improving conduct disorder or associated factors like aggression. The most useful comparison would be with the earlier reported meta-analysis examining the effects of social skills training for students with LD (Forness & Kavale, 1996b). Across 52 studies including about 2,000 subjects similar with respect to age and IQ, the $\overline{ES}$ for social skills training was .21, almost the same as the .20 found in the present investigation. In both cases, training produced a modest 8-percentile-rank gain and a situation where the student with E/BD or LD would be better off than only 58% of students receiving no social skills training.

A number of difficulties may contribute to the modest effects found for social skills training for students with E/BD, and these parallel the explanations suggested for the limited effects of social skills training found for students with LD. For example, intensity of training may also be a limiting factor. In the case of social skills training for students with E/BD, the program, on average, lasted about 12 weeks with about $2\frac{1}{2}$ hours per week devoted to training. The question arises: Was sufficient time allocated to modify basic elements of social competence? Similarly, as was the case with LD, the majority of training programs used were designed specifically for research purposes, which makes it difficult to determine what was actually happening as a result of training.

In the case of social skills training for students with E/BD, sampling problems may also contribute to the modest outcomes. A majority of studies selected subjects on the basis of the presence or absence of specific social skill deficits, with E/BD being a more secondary consideration. In only about 25% of the studies were subjects selected primarily on E/BD criteria (federal SED or DSM) with social skill deficits being a secondary, but necessary, consideration. When subjects are selected primarily on the basis of social skill deficits, two problems are encountered: The extent to which a subject is "truly" E/BD becomes indeterminant, and the social skill deficits may be far more severe and consequently more resistant to treatment than "milder" deficits associated with the constellation of factors defining E/BD. Thus, the nature of the sampling makes it difficult to determine the effectiveness of training for the "typical" student with E/BD.

Another difficulty related to sampling involves possible confounding between E/BD and LD. For LD samples, it is possible that social skill deficits are accounted for primarily by a subset of students comorbid for psychiatric disorders (e.g., ADHD, conduct disorder, depression) (San Miguel, Forness, & Kavale, 1996). This assumption is supported by some findings showing few, if any, social skill deficits may be present in selected LD samples (e.g., Bay, 1985; Cartledge, Stupay, & Kaczala, 1986; Pullis, 1985). Thus, a subset of students classi-fied as LD might be more properly classified E/BD. For example, academic underachievement has been found to occur early in the ontogeny of conduct disorder (Patterson, DeBaryshe, & Ramsey, 1989) and, consequently, LD may not be the most appropriate classification because behavior problems are a primary manifestation. Without a clear definition of who is being trained, samples may become confounded and the effects of social skills training difficult to deter-mine.

In summary, the available literature did not offer compelling evidence about the efficacy of social skills training. It appears that social skills training has limited value in intervention programs designed for students with E/BD.

## Conclusion

Although a popular adjunct intervention, social skills training does not appear to promote enhanced social functioning in students with LD or E/BD. Two research domains investigating the efficacy of social skills training for these two special education populations revealed limited effectiveness. The obtained $\overline{ES}$ s for social skills training were quite similar. The Kavale et al. (1997) meta-analysis, which also included a synthesis of 64 single-subject studies investigating social skills training for students with E/BD, also

found only a modest training effect. Such evidence, taken together, provides confidence in questioning whether social skills training is worth the time and effort.

Social competence is of paramount importance for students with special needs, particularly beyond the school years when social skills may assume more importance than academic skills. Within the context of special education, social skills training as a "special" intervention revealed the modest effects ($\overline{ES}$ = .20) associated with other "special" practices (e.g., perceptual-motor training [$\overline{ES}$ = .08], modality instruction [ES = .14], psycholinguistic training [$\overline{ES}$ = .39]). An inherent difficulty with special interven-tions like social skills training is the fact that they deal with unobservable con-structs like peer relations (see Newcomb, Bukowski, & Pattee, 1993) and prosocial behavior (see Eisenberg, 1991). These constructs present a variety of unresolved conceptual and definitional issues that require resolution before training can be evaluated in an unencumbered manner.

There is some indication of larger treatment effects (e.g., Schneider & Byrne, 1985) as well as greater impact for specific types of training (e.g., Durlak, Fuhrman, & Lampman, 1991; Dush, Hirt, & Schroeder, 1989) in general education students, and such findings need to be investigated to determine why some social skills training fails to demonstrate the same efficacy within the context of special education. Until such complexities are better understood, social skills training programs must be approached with caution and their inclusion in a special education intervention package questioned.

# CHAPTER 6

# EVALUATING THE EFFECTIVENESS OF SPECIAL EDUCATION

Since the inception of special education, a variety of unique procedures designed to enhance student performance have been developed. These procedures would not be routinely used in a general education context and have almost come to define the nature of special education. With their development, questions about their efficacy also arose. The methods and techniques discussed in chapters 2–5 represent a number of these special interventions, but the quantitative syntheses presented do not paint an optimistic picture about their efficacy. A summary of the meta-analyses presented in chapters 2–5 is presented in Table 31.

The very modest effects found for most of the interventions appear to militate against a positive conclusion about their efficacy. To provide perspec-

tive, suppose that an $\overline{ES}$ of 1.00 is used as a yardstick since this $\overline{ES}$ represents the average achievement gain of the average student at the end of one year's worth of instruction in an academic domain. With an average gain of 1 year ($\overline{ES} = 1.00$) for the average student on achievement measures, the special education interventions reviewed do not appear impressive since, on average, the special education student would gain only about 2 months on such an achievement measure. With most special interventions revealing $\overline{ES}$ below .50, they thus represent less advantage than one-half year's worth of schooling. It would not be unreasonable to demand that special interventions accelerate the rate of academic gain expected from general education if students in special education are to

## Table 31. Summary of Meta-Analyses for Traditional Special Education Interventions

| Intervention | Number of Studies | Mean Effect Size | *SD* of Effect Size |
|---|---|---|---|
| Perceptual-motor training | 180 | .08 | .27 |
| Diet modification | 23 | .12 | .42 |
| Modality instruction | 39 | .14 | .28 |
| Social skills training—E/BD | 41 | .20 | .54 |
| Social skills training—LD | 52 | .21 | .68 |
| Psychotropic medication | 70 | .30 | .75 |
| Psycholinguistic training | 34 | .39 | .54 |
| Stimulant medication | 135 | .58 | .61 |

Note. *SD* = standard deviation. E/BD = emotional/behavioral disturbance. LD = learning disability.

eliminate the discrepancies in their educational performance.

The special interventions demonstrated effects that primarily ranged from negligible to small and, at best, medium using Cohen's (1988) classification of *ES* magnitude. None approached the large effects (.80 and above) that would be necessary to enhance performance at a rate that would accelerate a special education student towards grade-level performance. For special interventions, the obtained $\overline{ES}$s are not eloquent testimony to the efficacy of practices that have almost come to define special education. To provide perspective, consider that something as simple (setting aside financial considerations) as reducing class size in general education (for example, from 35 to 25) can enhance achievement with an $\overline{ES}$ of .31 (see Glass & Smith, 1979). That six of the eight interventions discussed did not produce the same magnitude of effect suggests that the efficacy of special practices defining special education must be called into question.

In evaluating the effectiveness of special education, another complication arises besides the modest $\overline{ES}$ magnitude, and this is also illustrated by again examining the data in Table 31. Besides the $\overline{ES}$ shown in the second column, the associated standard deviation *(SD)* is displayed in the third column; the *SD* is a measure of dispersion around the mean and represents an index of variability. When compared to the $\overline{ES}$, the *SD* reveal magnitudes sometimes two to three times greater; in every case, the intervention exhibited greater variability than effectiveness. If the two statistics are combined ($\overline{ES} \pm SD$), they form a theoretical expectation about the magnitude of intervention efficacy (see

Kaplan, 1964). Simple arithmetic using this theoretical representation reveals that special education practice may vary from negative to zero to positive over a wide range. Although these are merely theoretically possible values, it does demonstrate that special interventions are more variable than beneficial in their effects. This variability is not a hallmark of effective practice; the variability makes special education essentially indeterminate and, consequently, it would be difficult to provide other than an equivocal response about the effectiveness of special education.

As part of meta-analytic procedure, important study features (e.g., age, gender, IQ, socioeconomic status, severity level) are correlated with *ES*. If some correlations are significant, then it is possible to stipulate the existence of an important association or relation; for example, that psycholinguistic training would be most effective with a particular special education classification, or social skills training would be most effective at a particular age level. In performing the meta-analyses described, perhaps hundreds of correlations were calculated, but very few were significant, suggesting that the relationships were not of a magnitude permitting useful prediction; the effectiveness of special interventions is thus also unpredictable.

The findings from the meta-analyses for the special education interventions reviewed suggest that they do not conform to the parameters of "perfect" knowledge that is represented by a lawful set of input-output associations (i.e., do A in circumstance X and Y and do B in circumstance Z) (see Brodbeck, 1962). Instead, the interventions examined indicate that special education is best viewed as imperfect (i.e., unlawful) knowledge, and should not operate on the basis of prescriptive action, a single course of action over a variety of situations. Imperfect knowledge is also confounded by the fact that generalizations in the behavioral sciences tend to change over time (see Gergen, 1973) because of modifications in the values underlying perceptions of what is important and desirable (Eisner, 1979). Special education, at least in the form of the special practices reviewed, needs to be understood as an enterprise that is variable, indeterminate, unpredictable, unlawful, and value-laden (Kavale, 1987). Under such circumstances, it is little wonder that special education has not demonstrated unequivocal efficacy.

# Why Special Education May Not Be Effective

The modest effectiveness found for many special education interventions may be related to the fact that too much emphasis has been placed on the adjective *special*. In order to define its uniqueness, special education developed *special* interventions, but their very uniqueness cast them in the role of instant and simple solutions for the educational needs of special education students. The difficulty, however, is that the special practices have never fulfilled the promise of being either *the* solution or *the* answer. The meta-analytic findings demonstrate clearly that no claim can be made for any special education intervention having provided either *the* solution or *the* answer.

Special education has also failed to clarify and resolve a number of conceptual problems that mediate intervention effectiveness. By explicating these conceptual issues, it is possible to explain partially why intervention activities do not often produce the expected positive results.

## *Belief Systems*

The first conceptual problem relates to what is believed about certain interventions. The strong clinical tradition and historical roots of many special education interventions (e.g., perceptual-motor training, modality matched instruction) strongly influence perceptions about their efficacy. Any negative research evidence is dismissed as inconclusive; questions about efficacy never achieve closure and basic beliefs are not altered. A good example is the modality concept, where better than 9 out of 10 teachers surveyed believed that modality strengths and weaknesses should be considered, and that students learn best when instruction is modified to match individual modality patterns (Arter & Jenkins, 1977; Kavale & Reese, 1991).

Although the Kavale and Forness (1987) quantitative synthesis offered a negative evaluation of the modality model, it is important to note that many previous reviews (e.g., Arter & Jenkins, 1979; Larrivee, 1981; Tarver & Dawson, 1978; Ysseldyke, 1973) reached similar conclusions. Nevertheless, because of the strong intuitive appeal associated with the modality model, the consistent and persistent negative evaluations are discounted in favor of unsubstantiated claims capitalizing on that intuitive appeal. Unlike old soldiers, the modality model does not fade away, as evidenced by yet another cycle of debate about its efficacy (see Carbo, 1992; Snider, 1992a, 1992b).

The strength of such belief is seen in Swanson's (1984) finding of a significant discrepancy between what teachers say and what they do. Teachers are apparently most comfortable with what they already know, what they have been exposed to, and what the conventional wisdom says. Regardless of how exciting teachers may find new theoretically based strategies, they tend to resist implementing them in favor of existing practices they find comfortable. Thus, a strong theoretical rationale does not appear to guide actual teaching practice.

## *Nonproductive Issues*

A second problem surrounds the nonproductive ways in which issues have come to be perceived. A prime example here is the concept of individualized instruction, the cornerstone of most special education models. In its classic sense as embodied in diagnostic-prescriptive teaching (see Peter, 1965), nothing is more fundamental to special education intervention than the idea that a student should be assessed to determine strengths and weaknesses and then instruction designed to capitalize on strengths and remediate weaknesses. Although seemingly uncontentious, the basic idea of diagnostic-prescriptive teaching has become contorted and polarized into diametrically opposed theoretical models (see Quay, 1973). For example, Ysseldyke and Salvia (1974) discussed the process (ability) model, where the goal is to identify processes that are strong or weak in order to prescribe remediation for the process deficits themselves with interventions like those described in chapter 3, versus the skill (behavioral) model, where the goal of task analysis is to assess academic skill development and design instruction to foster skill acquisition. The skill model emphasizes component skills and their integration rather than the training of

processes that presumably underlie skill development. In reality, neither model is satisfactory by itself (see Smead, 1977), and the primary effect of such philosophical debate is to deflect attention away from actual instructional practice.

Lloyd (1984) emphasized a similar point in an analysis of individualized instruction and its embodiment in aptitude-treatment interactions (ATI). Characteristics or aptitudes of certain students will interact with certain kinds of instructional programs or treatments in such a way that the students will learn better than if they had all been given one or the other treatment. The concept of ATI is central for individualized instruction in special education and is found in three models: (a) remedial—a particular treatment is provided to remedy impediments to student learning; (b) compensatory—a particular treatment will compensate for gaps in student knowledge or skill; and (c) preferential—particular treatments will match with a student's preferred style of learning, like the modality meta-analysis discussed in chapter 3 (see Salomon, 1972). Lloyd (1987) analyzed the three models and concluded that there was little empirical support for any of these aptitude x treatment interaction hypotheses. It was concluded that the assumption that some kinds of instruction are better for some students while other kinds are better for other students may not be valid; instruction instead should be based on "skills students need to be taught" (p. 14), which represents the fundamental premise of diagnostic-prescriptive teaching.

Fuchs and Fuchs (1986) followed this suggestion with a call for systematic formative evaluation as the basis for individualization. Systematic formative evaluation focuses on ongoing evaluation and program modification to provide a basis through which individualized programs may be developed. The advantages of systematic formative evaluation include these: (a) It is an inductive, rather than deductive, approach to individualization and thus avoids the pitfalls of formulating a diagnosis before the relationship between learner characteristics and educational intervention is fully established; (b) it is based on more psychometrically acceptable measurement procedures; and (c) it possesses more ecological validity because of repeated measurement in the actual classroom setting. Thus, discussion about individualization can be useful if structured in productive ways, rather than obfuscating the concept through the creation of nonproductive issues.

### Confounding Issues

A third conceptual problem surrounds the confounding of issues. The primary example is the long-standing issue of *where* special education students should be educated. Kauffman (1993), however, suggested the necessity for "keeping place in perspective" (p. 7) primarily because of limited knowledge about how placement determines what is possible and what is probable with respect to instruction and educational outcomes. From neither historical analysis (e.g., MacMillan & Hendrick, 1993) nor evaluations of placement effects (e.g., Hallahan, Keller, McKinney, Lloyd, & Bryan, 1988) is it possible to conclude that location is the primary factor in producing special education outcomes. Of greater importance, however, is what actually happens instructionally and the types of interactions that transpire in the particular setting (Gottlieb, Alter, & Gottlieb, 1991). The *what* is thus of greater import than

the *where,* but in special education the argument has been primarily about placement options, at the expense of instructional options.

## The Question of Place in the Delivery of Special Education

The magnitude and longevity of debate surrounding the question of where special education students should be placed should not be underestimated. It has been a primary issue since the 1940s and has escalated into debate about the viability of special education as a distinct and separate place (see Fuchs & Fuchs, 1994). What is missing, however, is critical discussion about what happens, instructionally and socially, in special education settings. This leads to what Mitroff and Featheringham (1974) termed Type III error, asking the "wrong" question when you should have asked the "right" question. Too much emphasis has been placed on the merits of different settings when they have relatively little effect per se on whether or not special education is effective.

Efficacy studies of special education placement have a long history. Polloway (1984) identified five historical stages and discussed the major question and time frame associated with each:

1. Would special education students profit from being in school together with nonhandicapped peers? (1930s to 1940s)

2. Are the needs of special education students best met in regular—or special—class programs? (1950s to mid 1960s)

3. Are special classes a viable program option for special education students

65

given the increasing legal, sociological, and political concerns as well as the paucity of research documenting their benefits? (late 1960s to early 1970s)

4. Given a variety of placement options within a "cascade" model of services, which alternative is most appropriate for the individual special education student? (early 1970s to 1980s)

5. Can the population of special education students benefit from the more integrated placements common since the passage of the Education for All Handicapped Act (PL 94-142)? (mid 1980s to present)

Although there is a long history of research investigating these questions, the findings have proved difficult to interpret and conclusions have been equivocal (e.g., Guskin & Spicker, 1968; Kirk, 1964; Meyers, MacMillan, & Yoshida, 1980). Nevertheless, legislation and litigation emphasized the "least restrictive environment" concept, and there has been a decided trend towards integration and primary placement in the general education class (Kavale, 1979). It is also important to note that advocacy for the mainstreaming movement was built primarily on ideological and philosophical arguments (e.g., Christopolos & Renz, 1969; Dunn, 1968) rather than empirical foundations, which suggests that the commitment to integration was more steadfast than warranted by the research evidence (MacMillan, 1971).

Carlberg and Kavale (1980) performed a meta-analysis on 50 studies examining the question of special class versus regular class placement. The 50 studies produced 322 $ES$ measurements and yielded an $\overline{ES}$ of .12. (The $ES$ statistic was arranged so that a positive $ES$ favored the special class while a negative $ES$ favored the regular or mainstreamed class.) These data represented approximately 27,000 students who averaged 11 years of age with a mean IQ of 74 and who remained in the special class for just under two years. Approximately 58% of the $ESs$ were negative: in more than half the cases, special classes were less effective than regular classes. Since the average comparison regular class subject would be at the 50th percentile, the effects of approximately two years of special class placement was to reduce the relative standing of the average special class subject by 5 percentile ranks. Thus, special class students were slightly worse off than if they had remained in regular classes.

Special education placement studies generally measured two outcomes. In the Carlberg and Kavale (1980) meta-analysis, achievement and social/personality variables revealed $\overline{ES}$ s of .15 and .11 respectively. Thus, special class placement was inferior to regular class placement on the two major outcomes measured; special class subjects declined by 6 and 4 percentile ranks on achievement and social/personality measures respectively. These findings lent support for a negative, albeit small, effect for special class placement suggesting that special class placement produced no tangible benefits. In practical terms, however, the transformation of this negative $\overline{ES}$ suggests that the average loss due to special class placement over approximately *two* years was only about 1 or 2 *months* of academic achievement, a relatively negligible outcome. Thus, special class placement was only slightly less efficacious than regular class placement and the question of place remains unanswered conclusively.

By the late 1970s, integration and the concept of mainstreaming came to be defined primarily by the resource model of service delivery (e.g., Deno, 1973; Hammill & Wiederholt, 1972; Reger, 1973). A resource program represents a structure where a teacher has responsibility for providing supportive educationally related service to special education students during specified time periods. An integral component is also a place, the resource room, where students receive specific instruction on a regularly scheduled basis, while receiving the majority of their education in a general education program.

By the mid-1980s, the resource model became the most frequently used special education service provision, particularly for students with high-incidence mild disabilities (Friend & McNutt, 1984). Although the resource model continued to develop (e.g., McLoughlin & Kelly, 1982; Speece & Mandell, 1980; Wiederholt, Hammill, & Brown, 1974), evaluations revealed considerable variability in outcomes and equivocal conclusions about efficacy (Sindelar & Deno, 1978; Wiederholt & Chamberlain, 1989).

Wang and Baker (1985–86) performed a meta-analysis on 52 studies investigating the efficacy of mainstreaming defined as placements in settings other than the special class. The analysis included 3,413 students across grades K–12 and across special education categories. The 52 studies produced 455 *ES* measurements and yielded an $\overline{ES}$ of .11 with about 40% negative *ES*. The $\overline{ES}$ of .11 indicates that 54% of mainstreamed students would be better off than those in comparison groups. For comparisons involving mainstreamed versus nonmainstreamed special

education students, the $\overline{ES}$ was .43, indicating that 67% of mainstreamed students were better off by about 17 percentile ranks as a result of a more integrated placement. When, however, the comparison group was nonhandicapped peers, the mainstreaming $\overline{ES}$ was .31, meaning that mainstreamed students lost 12 percentile ranks. There was a positive, albeit small, effect favoring mainstreamed settings; special education students in integrated programs outperformed those in self-contained settings but performed lower than their nonhandicapped peers.

The findings from meta-analyses investigating special education placements suggested only a modest effect on outcomes for different settings. By conventional standards (see Cohen, 1988), the obtained $\overline{ES}$ s, in all cases, were quite modest. The emphasis on setting brought about by the implementation of the cascade model (see Deno, 1970) with its continuum of placement options has made "place" the focus of attention (e.g., Leinhardt & Pallay, 1982); yet, little advantage was found for any placement, as evidenced by the small $\overline{ES}$ associated with outcome evaluations in different settings. Two explanations for the findings are possible: (a) Special education in any setting may indeed be ineffective, or (b) the methodology for studying the efficacy of special education in different places may not be appropriate. Analyses of the efficacy research have revealed a number of methodological difficulties that threaten the validity of findings (see Tindal, 1985), including these:

1. *Placement histories.* Different placements in a student's school history may interact with the student's current placement; the effect associated with each

67

successive intervention may become confounded with its order in the placement sequence (Cegelka & Tyler, 1970). Such confounded effects may limit generalizability of findings (see Campbell, 1969).

2. *Subject selection and assignment.* When sampling is not random, groups may not be comparable, and it is difficult to determine whether outcomes are related to treatment; consequently, internal validity is affected adversely (Campbell & Stanley, 1966; Cook & Campbell, 1979). Many studies of placement have not used random assignment of subjects to different settings but instead used existing groups that were probably not established on a random basis. Thus, group differences may be due to antecedent conditions rather than any effects of intervention (Kaufman & Alberto, 1976).

3. *Appropriateness of measurement.* Standardized tests may not be sensitive enough to detect small changes sometimes produced by intervention programs (Sheehan & Keogh, 1984). Additionally, tests, although purporting to measure similar skills, may not be interchangeable because very different behaviors may be sampled (Jenkins & Pany, 1978). Finally, most studies using standardized tests have reported findings in grade-equivalent scores, which have been found to possess a number of technical problems that limit their usefulness in interpreting outcomes (Berk, 1984).

4. *Low statistical power.* In statistical terms, power refers to the ability of statistical tests to detect significant treatment differences; the higher the power, the more sensitive the statistical test (Cohen, 1988). Power is not a function of the statistical test itself but rather is related to experimental design and data quality. For example, if the variability among different classroom mean outcomes is great relative to the variability among individual students, then the test has high power. Conversely, power is low when variability among different classroom mean outcomes is small relative to variability among students.

5. *Variability among definitions.* Studies of special education placement, although focusing on particular categories of special education, in reality investigate heterogeneous groups of students who have been classified according to diverse and often ambiguous criteria that may vary significantly across settings. Students classified into one category in one setting are likely to be different from those similarly identified in another setting (Hallahan & Kauffman, 1977). The reliance on categorical labels may thus limit the kinds of conclusions that may be drawn from efficacy research (Heller, Holtzman, & Messick, 1982).

Although it is difficult to draw conclusions related to categories of special education, some general conclusions may be possible, as evidenced in the Carlberg and Kavale (1980) meta-analysis. Besides calculating overall efficacy ($\overline{ES} = .12$), it was also possible to aggregate *ES* measurements into three special education classifications: mental retardation (MR) (IQ 50-75), slow learner (SL) (IQ 75-90), and learning disability (LD) or emotional or behavior disorder (E/BD). These findings are shown in Table 32.

Special class placement was most disadvantageous for special education students whose problem was lower IQ levels (MR and SL). In comparison to general education counterparts, SL students lost 13 percentile ranks while students with MR declined by 6 percentile ranks. For students with LD or E/BD in special classes, however, an improvement of 11 percentile ranks was associated with placement. The average student with LD or E/BD in a special class was thus better off than 61% of those who remained in a general education class.

The $\overline{ES}$ s for special education classification exceeded those found overall for outcomes and thus deserve attention. The most fundamental question is why some students (i.e., MR and SL) placed in special classes were slightly worse off than they would have been had they remained in a general education classroom. The significant variable would appear to be intelligence and how it relates to teacher expectation: The fact that a student is placed in a special class because of a low IQ may lower teacher expectations about performance and result in less effort on the teacher's part and less learning on the student's (see Rosenthal & Jacobson, 1968; Rosenthal & Rubin, 1978). The lower expectancy, be it conscious or unconscious, may divert instructional efforts away from academic pursuits. Additionally, differences, for example, in the structure of the curriculum and the nature of the outcome assessments may make the special class a place whose goal is primarily maintenance. Consequently, the special class may function as an instrument for preserving existing educational and social order, and not necessarily an arrangement for providing enhanced educational opportunities for special education students.

On the other hand, the average intelligence of students with LD and E/BD (at least, by definition) may not dampen teacher expectation. Teachers in special classes may take a more optimistic view of these students and strive to provide significant efforts aimed at improving academic functioning. Perhaps these efforts represent the "real" special education, not a system seeking the *status quo* but a system focusing upon individual learning needs and abilities in order to design the most effective program of *academic* remediation necessary to overcome *academic* deficits.

In summary, basic questions about the best placement option for special education students are complex and not easily answered. It seems evident that statements like, "There is no compelling body of evidence that segregated special education programs have significant benefit for students" (Gartner & Lipsky, 1987, p. 131) are not entirely warranted, and statements about particular placements cannot be so definitive. The studies of special education placement have included a number of service delivery

## Table 32. Average Effect Size by Special Education Classification for Special Versus Regular Class Placement

| Diagnosis | Average Effect of Special vs. Regular Placement | Number of Effect Sizes |
| --- | --- | --- |
| Moderate mental retardation (IQ 50–75) | −.14 | 249 |
| Slow learner (IQ 75–90) | −.34 | 38 |
| Learning disability or emotional/behavioral disturbance | .29 | 35 |

options and, since no service arrangement has proved more effective, it appears that outcome differences are related to indeterminate and imperceptible variables not easily assessed or controlled. As MacMillan (1971) noted some 25 years ago, "The real issue is not whether special classes or regular classes are better but rather where the best interests of the students might be" (p. 9), and this statement remains just as valid today. A basic problem seems to be that debate has focused on placement to such an extent that setting has come to be equated with treatment itself (Epps & Tindal, 1988). Clearly, setting is not the salient variable that determines academic success; as an independent variable, setting provides little insight into what may constitute effective instruction (Burstein & Guiton, 1984). For example,

variations in classroom environment factors accounted for almost 25% of the variance in the social acceptance or rejection of students with MR by their peers. Active involvement of students in teacher-directed instruction and cooperative learning that promoted interaction with nonhandicapped peers were associated with better outcomes (Slavin, 1991). The findings related to special education placement may, in fact, indicate the lack of differences between special and general education at the level of instruction. Features of instruction are probably the major influence on outcomes, but these are not unique to setting. Setting is thus a macrovariable; the real question becomes one of examining what happens in that setting (Maher & Bennett, 1984).

# CHAPTER 7

# EFFECTIVE INTERVENTION PRACTICES AND SPECIAL EDUCATION

The methods and techniques reviewed earlier emphasized the *special* aspect of special education; they were interventions that would be found only in special education and not usually used in general education. The meta-analytic findings, however, suggested only modest effectiveness for a majority of practices that were developed to define the nature of special education. In addition to these unique and singular interventions, special education has also developed interventions that emphasize the *education* part of special education. Over time, there has been less stress in special education on developing techniques aimed at enhancing the more hypothetical constructs associated with learning and more emphasis on methods that feature more substantive aspects of learning by adapting general education techniques for the purposes of special education.

Hagin (1973) reviewed intervention methods in special education and noted a shift in emphasis. Early efforts, prior to 1965, viewed the problems of special education students from a pathology perspective; academic disability was regarded as a disease entity, and interventions (e.g., perceptual-motor training) were aimed at removing the pathology. After 1965, emphasis shifted to what was termed an "educational mismatch model," where school failure was viewed as the result of a mismatch between educational methods and a student's developmental level. The educational mismatch model was gradually replaced (by about 1980) with a "learning process model" that was concerned with substantive aspects of

learning, particularly as they related to cognitive, linguistic, and social factors. Special education thus slowly shifted its emphasis from *special* to *education*. A number of quantitative research syntheses have assessed the effectiveness of interventions emphasizing *education*, and a review of these meta-analyses will be useful for comparisons with *special* interventions.

## Improving Reading Comprehension

For special education students with high-incidence mild disabilities (e.g., LD, MR), reading difficulties often represent the primary academic problem area. The reading problems often include a failure to recognize words and associate them with concepts, or a failure to recognize and interpret sentences that prevents the creation of a representation of the text and, ultimately, a failure to comprehend text (Perfetti, 1985). Although special education students were more likely to receive interventions aimed at enhancing decoding skills (e.g., Gillingham & Stillman, 1968), there has been increasing recognition that reading comprehension skills also need to be taught (Ysseldyke, Thurlow, O'Sullivan, & Christenson, 1989).

In response to the need of special education students for reading comprehension instruction, a number of techniques were developed. The array of interventions might include cognitive interventions (e.g., specific problem-solving skills, advanced organizers, approaching text with specific schema or rules, teaching students to remember specific facts), cognitive-behavioral interventions (e.g., self-monitoring behavior during reading, self-questioning about text), vocabulary interventions (e.g., correcting oral reading errors, pronunciation and meaning of words in isolation and context), pre- and mid-reading interventions (e.g., story previews, questions about the story), and direct instruction interventions (e.g., programmed materials, rapid oral responding, continuous evaluation and correction of inaccurate responding, teacher praise for attending and responding).

To determine the effectiveness of reading comprehension interventions for students with learning disabilities, Talbott, Lloyd, and Tankersley (1994) performed a meta-analysis on the findings from 48 studies representing 1,500 students with average IQ levels and an average age of 13 years, who received about 30 hours of reading comprehension instruction. Across 255 *ES* measurements, the $\overline{ES}$ was 1.13, indicating that the average special education student receiving a reading comprehension intervention scored at the 87th percentile on an outcome measure. Thus, a student receiving one of these interventions was better off than 87% of students not receiving a special reading comprehension intervention.

In a similar meta-analysis, Mastropieri, Scruggs, Bakken, and Whedon (1996) reviewed 68 studies investigating reading comprehension interventions for students with learning disabilities that included 2,865 students who averaged 13 years of age with an average IQ of 94 and who received about 7 $^1/_2$ hours of reading comprehension

instruction. The $\overline{ES}$ across 205 *ES* measurements was .98, which, in relative terms, translates into raising the performance of the average special education student from the 50th percentile to the 84th percentile on an outcome measure. As a result of reading comprehension instruction, the average trained subject was better off than 84% of subjects not receiving this special instruction.

The similar findings furnished by two independent investigations of attempts to enhance reading comprehension provide verification for concluding that the real effect is about 1 *SD* ($\overline{ES}$ = 1.00). The reliability of findings is further confirmed by the similar $\overline{ES}$ found for specific methods in the two meta-analyses. The findings are shown in Table 33. In both investigations, metacognitive (e.g., self-questioning, self-monitoring) methods produced the largest effects. Text enhancement procedures (e.g., advanced organizers, computer assistance, mnemonics) were the second most effective methods. Differences were noted for skill training procedures (e.g., vocabulary, repeated readings) and direct instruction procedures, but the differences amounted to only 5 percentile ranks. The consistency of the findings from these two independent meta-analyses provides confidence for concluding that it is possible to enhance the reading comprehension ability of students with learning disabilities.

The average general education student, after one year of instruction in reading comprehension, would show an $\overline{ES}$ of 1.00. Based on the two meta-analyses investigating teaching reading comprehension to students with learning disabilities, the obtained $\overline{ES}$ was 1.06, a level comparable to one year's worth of reading comprehension instruction. Thus, the special methods designed to enhance reading comprehension for students with learning disabilities produced the same effect as one year's worth of general education instruction ($\overline{ES}$ = 1.00) in approximately 18 hours; special education students can thus enhance the rate at which they improve their ability to better comprehend what they read.

# Mnemonic Instruction

With the recognition that many special education students possess memory deficits as a primary characteristic (e.g., Torgesen & Kail, 1980), efforts were directed at improving memory through the use of elaborative learning strategies. Since many memory deficits are language based (e.g., Kail & Leonard, 1986; Torgesen & Goldman, 1977; Vellutino & Scanlon, 1982), the goal is to enhance the representation of words in memory through training in more purposive information-processing strategies. One such strategy is mnemonic training, which attempts to transform difficult-to-remember facts into a more memorable form (Mastropieri & Scruggs, 1991). A common method is the keyword approach, which reconstructs unfamiliar verbal stimuli into acoustically similar representations and elaborates the reconstructed stimuli with response information (Atkinson, 1975). For example, in the domain of science, to teach that the mineral *apatite* is No. 5 on Moh's hardness scale, is *brown* in color, and is used for making *fertilizer*, students are first taught a "key word" for apatite, a familiar concrete word that is orthographically or phonetically similar. In this case, *ape* is the key word. Then, students are taught rhyming "peg words" for recalling the numbers 1 through 10 (e.g., 1 is *bun*, 2 is *shoe*, 3 is *tree)*. In the case of apatite, 5 is *hive*. Finally, students are shown an interactive illustration of a *brown ape* pouring a bag of *fertilizer* on a *beehive*. Students are thus provided with a direct retrieval route for all factual information associated with the mineral apatite.

The method capitalizes on the three "mnemonic R's" (Levin, 1983): (a) *recoding*, where the unfamiliar stimulus term is recoded into a more familiar, concrete proxy (e.g., apatite = ape); (b) *relating*, where the recoded stimulus is

## Table 33. Effects of Reading Comprehension Instructional Methods

| Method | Mean Effect Size | |
| --- | --- | --- |
| | Talbott et al.[a] | Mastropieri et al.[b] |
| Metacognitive | 1.60 | 1.33 |
| Text enhancement | 1.09 | .92 |
| Skill training (e.g., vocabulary) | .79 | .62 |
| Direct instruction | .67 | .81 |
| Overall | 1.13 | .98 |

[a]Talbott, Lloyd, & Tankersley, 1994. [b]Mastropieri, Scruggs, Bakken, & Whedon, 1996.

related to the to-be-learned information via an interactive episode (e.g., a picture of a brown ape pouring fertilizer over a hive); and (c) *retrieving*, where the learner is provided with a direct retrieval route from the stimulus (apatite) to all associated information (brown, 5, fertilizer). Mnemonic instruction has proved effective for teaching vocabulary (e.g., Mastropieri, Scruggs, & Fulk, 1990; Mastropieri, Scruggs, Levin, Gaffney, & McLoone, 1985; Scruggs, Mastropieri & Levin, 1985) and science information (e.g., Scruggs, Mastropieri, Levin, & Gaffney, 1985; Scruggs, Mastropieri, McLoone, Levin, & Morrison, 1987). Additionally, mnemonic instruction has been successfully incorporated into existing curricular materials through a model of "reconstructive elaborations," where to-be-learned content is reconstructed along the dimensions of meaningfulness and concreteness and linked with stimulus and response information for the student (Mastropieri & Scruggs, 1991). Through the use of acoustic, symbolic, and mimetic reconstructions, content area information has been successfully adapted for classroom use (e.g., Mastropieri, Scruggs, Whittaker, & Bakken, 1994; Scruggs & Laufenberg, 1986; Scruggs & Mastropieri, 1989, 1992).

Mastropieri and Scruggs (1989) synthesized the experimental literature investigating the effectiveness of mnemonic instruction with special education students using meta-analytic procedures. Across 19 studies and 983 subjects, the $\overline{ES}$ was 1.62, indicating that the average special education student receiving mnemonic instruction would be better off than 95% of students not receiving such instruction. The expected 45-percentile-rank gain on an outcome

assessment means that special education students may almost double their original scores when instructed mnemonically. The associated standard deviation (.79) is also noteworthy because it indicates the presence of no negative effects (i.e., control subjects outperforming experimental subjects). The uniformly positive effects (range = .68 to 3.42) for mnemonic instruction suggest that it represents an effective means for enhancing the academic performance of special education students.

# Direct Instruction

Direct instruction is usually represented through a set of behaviorally oriented teaching procedures. The term began as a general description of effective teaching behaviors (e.g., Rosenshine, 1976) and moved to a more comprehensive view that included not only effective instruction but also curriculum design, classroom management, and teacher preparation (Gersten, Woodward, & Darch, 1986). The term became formalized as *direct instruction* (DI) (Engelman & Carnine, 1982; Gersten & Keating, 1987), a prescriptive set of instructional materials that are scripted for teachers so as to insure that effective teaching behaviors are incorporated into individual lessons. DI is the basis for programs like *Reading Mastery: DISTAR Reading* (Engelman & Bruner, 1988) and *Corrective Reading Program* (Engelman, Becker, Hanner, & Johnson, 1988). Each program is structured around six critical features (see Gersten, Carnine, & Woodard, 1987):

1. An explicit step-by-step strategy.

2. Development of mastery at each step in the process.

3. Strategy (or process) corrections for student errors.

4. Gradual fading from teacher-directed activities toward independent work.

5. Use of adequate systematic practice with a range of examples.

6. Cumulative review of newly learned concepts.

White (1988), using the methods of meta-analysis, synthesized 25 studies investigating the effectiveness of DI and found an $\overline{ES}$ of .84. Special education students taught with DI procedures would be better off than 80% of students taught with comparison instructional methods and would be expected to gain about 30 percentile ranks on an outcome measure as a result of DI. Reading and math outcome assessments revealed $\overline{ES}$s of .85 and .50, respectively. Although the total $\overline{ES}$ for reading was comparable to the overall $\overline{ES}$ (.84), DI was less effective for the specific reading skills of word attack ($\overline{ES} = .64$) and reading comprehension ($\overline{ES} = .54$). Nevertheless, DI appears to result in an approximate 11-percentile-rank advantage for reading over math. Although not uniformly positive (14% negative $ES$), DI appears to be a useful teaching technique for enhancing the academic performance of students in special education.

# Peer Tutoring

The use of students as instructional agents has a long history (e.g., Allen, 1976), and a variety of academic and social benefits have been suggested for both tutor and tutee as a result of such pairing (e.g., Delquadri, Greenwood, Whorton, Carta, & Hall, 1986). For tutors, the academic benefits often include learning more than tutees while the social benefits may include a more positive attitude about school, increased responsibility, improved self-esteem, and greater self-confidence (see Scruggs & Richter, 1985). For special education, tutoring may provide the basis for delivering the individualized instruction that is the cornerstone of intervention.

Cook, Scruggs, Mastropieri, and Casto (1985–86) performed a meta-analysis on 19 studies investigating the effects of tutoring. The average investigation included 19 subjects who were 12 years old and were involved in 11 hours of tutoring over 29 sessions where each lasted for 25 minutes. Across 54 comparisons, tutors showed an $\overline{ES}$ of .53 and tutees an $\overline{ES}$ of .58, suggesting a better than one-half $SD$ advantage for both tutors and tutees above their respective comparison groups. For academic outcomes, tutees displayed greater $\overline{ES}$ gains than tutors on reading (.49 vs. .30), math (.85 vs. .67), and language (1.13 vs. .25) outcome measures.

On measures of attitude towards school and other students, the $\overline{ES}$ was higher for tutees (.86) than for tutors (.25). For self-concept and sociometric measures, negligible effects were found for both tutors and tutees. Behavior ratings, where tutors displayed larger $\overline{ES}$ than tutees (.89 vs. .10), suggest that tutors were perceived to change more than tutees.

Thus, peer tutoring programs for students in special education appear to be effective for both tutors and tutees. Tutees demonstrated greater achievement gains and more positive attitudes while tutors revealed more positive behavior changes. These findings generally conform to findings for tutoring involving general education students (e.g., Cohen, Kulik, & Kulik, 1982) and suggest that tutoring efforts in special education produces similar academic and social gains.

# Computer-Assisted Instruction

Advances in technology have resulted in increased use of computer-assisted instruction (CAI) to enhance educational performance. Generally, CAI has been found advantageous in general education (e.g., Niemic, Samson, Weinstein, & Walberg, 1987), and CAI has also been incorporated into special education programs and classrooms (e.g., Budoff, Thormann, & Gras, 1984; Lewis, 1993). The potential advantages for special education students include individualization and self-pacing, immediate feedback, consistent correction procedures, well-sequenced instruction, repetition without pressure, and increased time on task (Vockell & Mihail, 1993). The use of CAI may take a variety of forms including tutorials, guided practice, games, simulations, problem solving, and discovery learning (Malouf, Jamison, Kercher, & Carlucci, 1991) CAI has been shown to be useful for instruction in reading, math, writing, and critical thinking (e.g., Lieber & Semmel, 1985).

The use of CAI with special education students was investigated by Schmidt, Weinstein, Niemic, and Walberg (1985–86) in a meta-analysis of 26 studies. Of the 26 studies, 23 showed positive findings, and across 48 $ES$ measurements, the $\overline{ES}$ was .67. The average special education student would thus gain about 25 percentile ranks with CAI and be better off than 75% of students not receiving CAI. The application of CAI in special education appears to be effective, and, although some caution has been urged (e.g., Cosden & Abernathy, 1990; Goldman & Pellegrino, 1987), CAI can be recommended as an integral component in educational planning for students in special education (Thormann, Gersten, Moore, & Morvant, 1986).

# Formative Evaluation

Although not a specific method like, for example, DI, formative evaluation, the ongoing evaluation and modification of instructional procedures, has been suggested as a useful technique for enhancing the effectiveness of special instruction. Fuchs and Fuchs (1986) proposed the use of systematic formative evaluation for designing individualized programs that can overcome many of the difficulties found in the search for aptitude x treatment interactions (ATI), the method most often used for individualizing instruction (see Lloyd, 1984). Fuchs and Fuchs suggested that "this approach employs regular monitoring of handicapped students' performance under different instructional procedures. The purpose of this monitoring is to provide a data base with which individualized programs may be developed empirically" (1986, p. 200).

Fuchs and Fuchs (1986) found 21 studies investigating the effects of systematic formative evaluation. Using the methods of meta-analysis, an $\overline{ES}$ of .70 was found, indicating that the upper 50% of the experimental group exceeded about 76% of the control group. The effect of systematic formative evaluation (in conjunction with instruction) would thus raise an achievement outcome from the 50th to the 76th percentile. Although no differences were found with respect to age, treatment duration, frequency of measurement, or diagnostic classification, there were larger effects associated with behavior modification (reinforcement) in conjunction with systematic formative evaluation ($\overline{ES}$ = 1.12), with the employment of explicit, systematic data evaluation rules rather than teacher judgment in decisions about instructional changes ($\overline{ES}$ = .91), and with methods that required data to be graphed rather then simply recorded ($\overline{ES}$ = .70).

The findings suggest that systematic formative evaluation can reliably enhance the academic performance of students in special education. Although some objection to systematic formative evaluation has been lodged on the basis of its time-consuming nature (e.g., Wesson, King, & Deno, 1984), the magnitude of effect ($\overline{ES}$ = .70) produced by the procedure appears to warrant its use on a "cost-benefit" basis. As opposed to methods of individualized instruction that rely on deductive formulations, systematic formative evaluation is an inductive approach that appears to result in successful individualized programs.

# Behavior Modification

Skiba and Casey (1985), using the methods of meta-analysis, investigated the efficacy of applied behavior analysis techniques in enhancing academic and behavioral outcomes of students in special education. Across 41 studies, a total of 26 *ES* measurements produced an $\overline{ES}$ of .93, indicating nearly a 1-*SD* advantage for special education students.

In the behavioral area, an $\overline{ES}$ of .77 was found, indicating that the average special education student in a behavior modification program would demonstrate about a 28-percentile-rank gain on a behavioral outcome measure. Classroom behavior ($\overline{ES}$ = .93) improved more than social interaction ($\overline{ES}$ = .69). The average student in special education would thus be better off than 94% and 75%, respectively, of comparison students

with respect to classroom behavior and social interaction.

In the academic area, an $\overline{ES}$ of 1.57 was found when intervention targeted basic achievement skills. This effect amounts to about a 44-percentile-rank gain on an achievement measure and indicates that about 94% of the special education students would be better off than comparison group students not receiving applied behavior analysis interventions. The robust $\overline{ES}$ (.93) found by Skiba and Casey (1985) was confirmed in the Fuchs and Fuchs (1986) meta-analysis where a large $\overline{ES}$ (1.12) was found for behavior modification techniques when used in conjunction with formative evaluation. Thus, behavior modification appears to be a powerful intervention technique, especially when used to enhance academic skills.

# Early Intervention

Beginning with the Iowa studies (Skeels & Dye, 1939), there has been interest in early intervention to reduce the negative effects of disabilities or to prevent the development of learning and developmental problems in children presumed to be at risk for such problems. A number of investigations reported positive outcomes for early intervention (e.g., Gray, Ramsey, & Klaus, 1982; Kirk, 1958; Shonkoff & Hauser-Cram, 1988). Additionally, large-scale studies like the Perry Preschool project (Schweinhart, Berrueta-Clement, Barnett, Epstein, & Weikart, 1985), the Milwaukee project (Garber, 1988), the Juniper Gardens project (Greenwood et al., 1992), Carolina Abecedarian project (Martin, Ramey, & Ramey, 1990), and the Infant Health and Development Program (Ramey et al., 1992) have demonstrated that benefits accrue from early intervention programs. Although findings have generally been positive, several methodological problems has made it difficult to draw unequivocal conclusions (e.g., Odom & Karnes, 1988; Ramey & Ramey, 1992; White, Bush, & Casto, 1986).

Casto and Mastropieri (1986), using meta-analysis procedures, synthesized the findings from 74 studies investigating the effectiveness of early intervention. Across 215 *ES* measurements, the $\overline{ES}$ was .68, suggesting that a child enrolled in an early intervention program could be expected to gain about 25 percentile ranks on a variety of IQ, motor, language, and academic achievement outcome assessments. Thus, a child receiving early intervention was better off than 75% of children not enrolled in such a program.

A number of other variables were analyzed by Casto and Mastropieri (1986). Level of parent participation was not a major factor related to intervention success. Minor (or no) parent participation actually produced a larger $\overline{ES}$ (.76) than situations were parents played a major (or sole) role in the program ($\overline{ES}$ = .54). With respect to age at which intervention begins, the idea that "earlier is better" was not supported. Interventions that began when a child was 6–18 months of age were less effective ($\overline{ES}$ = .48) than programs begun when a child was 36–48 months of age ($\overline{ES}$ = 1.06). The child 6–18 months of age receiving early intervention would be expected to move from the 50th to the 68th percentile compared to a move to the 86th percentile for a child first enrolled at 36–48 months of age. Degree of program structure showed no difference, and any degree of structure produced an approximate 30-percentile-rank advantage. The intensity of intervention appeared to be an important factor. Interventions lasting 500 hours or more ($\overline{ES}$ = .86) and

including more than 10 hours per week ($\overline{ES}$ = .80) produced larger effects than, for example, interventions totaling less than 50 hours ($\overline{ES}$ = .56) with less than 2 hours per week ($\overline{ES}$ = .59).

In summary, early intervention appears to produce positive and robust effects. Programs that were longer and more intense produced even greater gains, while the conventional wisdom about age at start and degree of parental involvement was not supported. Thus, early intervention appears effective in enhancing the subsequent academic performance of special education students.

# Effective Special Education

The techniques and practices reviewed in this chapter are summarized in Table 34. When compared to the unique procedures that traditionally define special education (see Table 31), the interventions reviewed in this chapter paint a different picture of efficacy. The obtained effects demonstrated, at least, medium *ES* magnitude (i.e., .50) with a majority revealing large effects (i.e., .80 and above) based on Cohen's (1988) classification of *ES* magnitude. The students in special education receiving these interventions would be better off than 70% to 95% of students not receiving these interventions and would gain from 20 to 45 percentile ranks on an outcome assessment. On a standardized achievement test with a population mean of 100 and a standard deviation of 15, the use of the interventions listed in Table 34 would raise the average achievement score from 100 to anywhere from 108 to 124. For about half of the interventions reviewed, the effects parallel or exceed the benefits that accrue from one year's worth of instruction in general education ($\overline{ES}$ = 1.00). In all

## Table 34. Summary of Meta-Analyses for Effective Special Education Interventions

| Intervention | Number of Studies | Mean Effect Size | *SD* of Effect Size |
|---|---|---|---|
| Computer-assisted instruction | 22 | .52 | .33 |
| Peer tutoring | 19 | .56 | .69 |
| Early intervention | 74 | .67 | .73 |
| Formative evaluation | 21 | .70 | .53 |
| Direct instruction | 25 | .84 | .76 |
| Behavior modification | 41 | .93 | .48 |
| Reading comprehension | 82 | .98 | 1.05 |
| | 48 | 1.13 | 1.79 |
| Mnemonic strategies | 19 | 1.62 | .79 |

Note. *SD* = standard deviation.

cases, the benefits represent more advantage than one-half year of school and suggest that these interventions can successfully accelerate the rate of academic gain for special education students.

When considered in relation to the associated *SD,* the interventions summarized in Table 34 demonstrate less variability than the traditional interventions, where the *SD* revealed magnitudes sometimes two to three times greater than $\overline{ES}$ (see Table 31). For a majority of the interventions reviewed in this chapter, the *SD* was smaller than the $\overline{ES}$, and in no instance was it more than about 20% greater than $\overline{ES}$. Thus, the interventions shown in Table 34 appear to be more effective than variable, which means that instances of negative effects (i.e., comparison [control] students outperform special education students receiving the interventions) are unlikely. The limited variability makes these interventions far more determinate and, with the substantial magnitude of effect, permits a

positive response to questions about their efficacy.

## Special *Education* and *Special* Education

In a mega-analysis of special education interventions (the mean of all $\overline{ES}$), an $\overline{ES}$ of .54 was obtained (see Forness, Kavale, Blum, & Lloyd, 1997). Although 70% of students receiving these interventions would be better off by about 20 percentile ranks, an $\overline{ES}$ of .54 occupies an equivocal position between effectiveness and ineffectiveness. For some interventions, efficacy appears unequivocal while others reveal some promise. Finally, for other interventions, the evidence indicates that they should not be endorsed. Thus, taken as a whole, meta-analysis paints a variegated picture about special education efficacy that is likely to engender debate about its effectiveness.

Although judgments about the efficacy of special education remain equivocal in some cases, the findings from the meta-analyses indicated instances with far less equivocal findings. The contrasts revealed in Tables 31 and 34 suggest the possibility of terming some interventions effective (e.g., mnemonic training) and others ineffective (e.g., perceptual-motor training). Besides judgments about efficacy, it is also important to determine why some interventions are more effective than others. In examining the interventions reviewed, it seems that the variations in efficacy may be related, at a very fundamental level, to differences in the way the nature of special education is conceptualized.

The differences in conceptualization appear to be related to whether *special* or *education* is emphasized in special education. The interventions displayed in Table 31 appear to emphasize *special* by being unique and different methods that would not be routinely used in general education. For the most part, these interventions were designed solely for the purposes of special education with the goal of enhancing hypothetical and unobservable constructs that were presumably the cause of learning deficits. Education, in the form of acquisition of new knowledge, was secondary to improving skills and abilities that presumably underlie academic learning and need to be intact before more formal learning can occur. In contrast, the interventions displayed in Table 34 appear to emphasize *education* by adapting and modifying instruction. These interventions had their origin in general education and were transformed by special education to accommodate the needs of special education students. Education was a primary purpose; the enhanced acquisition and assimilation of content area knowledge was a major goal for these interventions. Rather than focusing on hypothetical constructs presumably related to learning ability, the interventions emphasizing *education* attempted a more direct approach by adapting instruction to enhance the academic learning of special education students.

The contrast between these two emphases is shown in Table 35, which compares methods of *special* (i.e., unique and different) education and special *education* (i.e., adapting and modifying instruction). The seven *special* education interventions produce an $\overline{ES}$ of .25, which means only about a 10% advantage for students receiving these interventions. For example, in the case of perceptual-motor training, the Feingold diet, modality instruction, and social skills training, the average special education student would gain only 3 to 8 percentile ranks on an outcome measure. On average, the upper 50% of the group receiving these special interventions exceeds only about 56% of the group not receiving such interventions; this modest level of improvement is only slightly above chance (50%). In addition, on average, about 25% of *ESs* for *special* education intervention were negative, indicating that in about 1 in 4 instances the student not receiving the *special* intervention did better on an outcome measure. Given the limited benefits, the wisdom of including *special* education interventions in a program is open to serious question.

In sharp contrast are interventions that can be termed special *education* and emphasize effective and validated instructional techniques. The seven interventions in this group produced an $\overline{ES}$ of .91. As a group, special *education* is almost 4 times as effective as *special* education, and is likely to move the

## Table 35. *Special* Education Versus Special *Education*

| *Special* Education | | Special *Education* | |
|---|---|---|---|
| Method | Mean Effect Size | Method | Mean Effect Size |
| Stimulant medication | .58 | Mnemonic strategies | 1.62 |
| Psycholinguistic training | .39 | Reading comprehension | 1.13 |
| Psychotropic medication | .30 | | .98 |
| Social skills training | .21 | Behavior modification | .93 |
| | .20 | Direct instruction | .84 |
| Modality instruction | .14 | Early intervention | .67 |
| Feingold diet | .12 | Peer tutoring | .56 |
| Perceptual-motor training | .08 | Computer-assisted instruction | .52 |
| Mean | .25 | | .91 |

average special education student from the 50th to the 82nd percentile. The 32-percentile-rank gain is better than 5 times the gain demonstrated from *special* education interventions and means that the average student would be better off than 82% of those not receiving special *education*. Even the smallest $\overline{ES}$ for special *education* (.52) is twice as effective as the average *special* education intervention (.25). Four special *education* practices produced gains comparable to one year's worth of schooling ($\overline{ES} = 1.00$), and two exceeded that level in a treatment period of about 20 days compared to the average 180-day school year. Even for interventions that employ a theoretical matching strategy, the more substantive mnemonic instruction ($\overline{ES} = 1.62$) was 10 times more effective than modality instruction ($\overline{ES} = .15$). Students in

special education, for example, who receive mnemonic instruction would be better off than 98% of students not receiving such instruction and would gain over $1^1/_2$ years of credit on an achievement measure compared to about 1 month for modality instruction. The evidence appears unequivocal: special education interventions that emphasize *education* over *special* are far more effective. When grounded in sound instructional methodology, special *education* can sometimes be up to 20 times more effective than *special* education practices that attempt to "cure" special education students by overcoming the negative effects on learning caused by a variety of hypothetical and unobservable constructs (e.g., modality and perceptual-motor factors).

# CHAPTER 8
# CREATING EFFECTIVE SPECIAL EDUCATION

Although some generalizations about the efficacy of special education seem possible, any such conclusions must remain tentative. A number of interventions were reviewed but not all. To attain a more comprehensive perspective, quantitative synthesis of other interventions should be undertaken. A variety of interventions emphasizing both *special* and *education* aspects of special education were not included here, and until the findings from other meta-analyses are included, the present conclusions should be approached with caution. The addition of other meta-analyses describing the effectiveness and variability of other interventions will provide a more complete picture about the efficacy of special education.

Even with the limitations imposed by not including all methods and techniques, the interventions compared and contrasted in this analysis suggest confidence in the conclusion that special education becomes significantly more effective when the *education* aspect is emphasized. It is evident that, when the *special* is emphasized, only modest outcomes are achieved and the outcomes reveal limited effectiveness. Enhanced effectiveness, however, becomes possible when special practices are based on sound instructional techniques. The goal then becomes one of adapting instructional procedures for the purposes of special *education*, and it would be useful to determine how this might be best accomplished.

The teaching-learning process, whether in general or special education, is enormously complex; learning has been shown to be mediated through a whole host of intervening variables (e.g., Dunkin & Biddle, 1974; Joyce & Weil, 1972; Peterson & Walberg, 1979). Beginning in the early 1980s, a number of factors were identified that influence school performance, and this body of research has come to be termed the "effective school" research (e.g., Mackenzie, 1983; Purkey & Smith, 1983; Squires, 1983).

Myriad findings about effective schooling practices have been shown to be strong and robust enough to warrant implementation as best practice (e.g., Haertel, Walberg, & Weinstein, 1983; Walberg, 1984; Waxman & Walberg, 1982). For special education in particular, Christenson, Ysseldyke, and Thurlow (1989) identified nine critical factors for positive instructional outcomes:

1. Classrooms are managed effectively.

2. There is a sense of positiveness in the school environment.

3. There is an appropriate instructional match.

4. Goals are clear, expectations are explicitly communicated, and lessons are presented clearly.

5. Students receive good instructional support.

6. Sufficient time is allocated to instruction.

7. Opportunity to respond is high.

8. Teachers actively monitor student progress.

9. Student performance is evaluated appropriately and frequently.

Similarly, Waxman, Wang, Anderson, and Walberg (1985) identified features of successful adaptive instruction for mainstream settings that include these factors:

1. An instructional match is maintained for each student.

2. Individualized pacing for achieving instructional goals is maintained.

3. Student progress is monitored, and continuous feedback is provided.

4. Students are involved in the planning and monitoring of their learning.

5. A broad range of techniques and materials are used.

6. Students help each other to learn.

7. Students are taught self-management skills.

8. Teachers engage in instructional teaming.

It is evident that much is known about what makes instruction effective. Although originating in general education, components of effective instruction have also been studied in special education, and much is known about such factors as motivation (Alderman, 1990), classroom management (Wang, 1987), providing success experiences (Reith & Evertson, 1988), establishing goals and expectations (Fuchs, Fuchs, & Deno, 1985), progress monitoring (Slavin & Madden, 1989), providing feedback (Larrivee, 1986), positive and supportive environments (Lovitt, 1984), teaching generalization (Ellis, Lenz, & Sabornie, 1987), and teaching independent learning skills (Pressley & Harris, 1990).

In examining the literature, it appears that the most investigated area is teacher behavior, to determine what factors produce a positive influence on student achievement (e.g., Brophy & Good, 1986; Medley, 1982; Weil & Murphy,

1982). For special education teachers, critical behaviors include these (Reith & Evertson, 1988):

1. Maintaining an academic focus in selecting activities and directing work.

2. Maintaining direction and control in the management of the learning environment.

3. Holding high expectations for academic progress.

4. Holding students accountable for satisfactory completion of work.

5. Having students work together cooperatively rather than competitively.

6. Establishing a positive affective climate.

The implementation of these positive teaching behaviors creates "active teaching" (Brophy & Good, 1986) where "the teacher carries the content to the students personally rather than depending on the curriculum to do so" (p. 361). The primary task of the teacher is to direct learning experiences, and "students spend most of their time being taught rather than working on their own (or not working at all)" (p. 361); this active teaching has been related to enhanced achievement. Stevens and Rosenshine (1981) stated, "Teachers who most successfully promoted achievement gain played the role of strong leader; that is, they selected and directed the academic activities, approached the subject matter in a direct, businesslike way, organized learning around questions they posed, and occupied the center of attention" (p. 2). The use of such systematic instructional procedures has also been supported in special education (Reynolds, Wang, & Walberg, 1992).

The implementation of direct and systematic instructional approaches creates the individualized instruction that is a cornerstone of special education (Talmage, 1975). Additionally, increased opportunity to learn is created which, in the form of academic learning time (ALT), is a major contributor to enhanced learning (Denham & Lieberman, 1980; Wilson, 1987). The amount of engaged time for general education students has been shown to be positively associated with learning (Fisher & Berliner, 1985) and is also a critical factor in the success of students in special education (Goodman, 1990), with findings showing that special education students require more time to achieve mastery (e.g., Gettinger, 1991; Greenwood, 1991). Wilson and Wesson (1986) suggested that instructional time, time on task, and student success are essential components of ALT in special education. They offered a number of suggestions to increase actual instructional time, time on task during teacher-directed instruction, and on-task behavior during practice. Thus, effective instruction is predicated on establishing appropriate academic instructional objectives and designing intervention programs that maximize opportunities for the special education student to work successfully on tasks related to those instructional objectives (Englert, Tarrant, & Mariage, 1992).

# Barriers to Effective Special Education

The research on effective schools and instruction has been studied in special education settings, and implications for special education have been described (e.g., Bickel & Bickel, 1986; Samuels, 1986). Essentially, it has been suggested that the valuable insights obtained about what makes general education instruction effective are also applicable to special education, but an "effective" school does not eliminate the need for special education. Although special education students achieved better academic and social outcomes in integrated programs at effective schools compared to those in special classes at equally effective schools, the special education students in integrated programs did more poorly than low-achieving but non-special-education peers (Deno, Maruyama, Espin, & Cohen, 1990). Generally, special education students achieved at levels below those attained by their low-achieving non-special-education peers with some indication of an inverse relationship between general education students' reading performance and that of special education students in effective schools (Semmel et al., 1994).

A number of investigations, however, have shown that discrepancies exist between the documented components of effective instruction and observations of actual special education practice (Morsink, Soar, Soar, & Thomas, 1986). In examining reading instruction in self-contained classrooms, for example, Leinhardt, Zigmond, and Cooley (1981) found that, while full days were allocated to reading, only about one-third of the day was actually spent reading. Similarly, Haynes and Jenkins (1986) found significant variability in the time students spent on direct reading; there was almost no relationship between student need and the time offered for actual reading in programs. The characteristics of special education students, particularly with respect to lower reading achievement levels, were found to be only weakly linked to scheduling and the amount of reading instruction received. Across content areas, for example, Englert (1983, 1984) demonstrated that only a relatively modest amount of time was spent on activities that could be considered direct instruction with active learner involvement and teacher attention. In general, Ysseldyke, Thurlow, Christenson, and Weiss (1987) reported that the percentage of engaged time in special education classes was about 75%, and that the amount of engaged time varied across classrooms as well as among individual students within a classroom.

It seems safe to conclude that there is wide variation in implementing the components of effective instruction. Good (1983) suggested that many teachers do not actively teach content; instruction consists of brief explanations followed by long periods of seatwork that do not provide sufficient opportunities for meaningful and successful practice. Brophy (1982) further suggested that the content of instruction defined in the curriculum is often the subject of deletions, additions, and incorrect applications when implemented by teachers in classrooms. The distortions due to teacher misinterpretations of content are more typical than any indirect distortion resulting from incomplete or inadequate teaching. Consequently, students may be presented content that is fragmented, limited, repetitive, and mystifying. Thus, general education may also not always follow the tenets of effective instruction.

Within the realm of special education, a number of research-based practices have been developed and shown to enhance academic functioning (see Mastropieri & Scruggs, 1994). Although these research-based special education practices are equally applicable for general education, there appears to be resistance to change in general education even when special education students are integral to the setting. This resistance is evidenced, for example, by undifferentiated large-group instruction being the norm, little deviation from the sequence of lessons outlined in teacher manuals, and little modification of content, pace, or grading criteria for special education students in general education settings (Vaughn & Schumm, 1996). A number of investigations (e.g., Baker & Zigmond, 1990; Fuchs, Fuchs, & Bishop, 1992; Nowacek, McKinney, & Hallahan, 1990) have demonstrated that the resources and assistance provided by special education have only marginal effects in general education contexts because of an entrenched refusal to incorporate positive instructional changes. On the other hand, Fuchs and Fuchs (1995a) have suggested that some general education practices (e.g., team teaching, collaborative consultation, cooperative learning) that have been offered as effective for educating special education students have really not been validated in either special or general education settings. In essence, all these findings suggest that generalizations about best practice are far from prescriptive at this point and further study is needed to determine where and how these practices are best implemented. The gap between theory and practice must be narrowed before it is possible to talk confidently about effective instruction—either general or special.

# Research, Evaluation, and Effective Instruction

The research base for describing effective instruction has long been predicated upon a basic process-product paradigm shown in Figure 3(a). The goal is to search for processes (teacher behaviors)

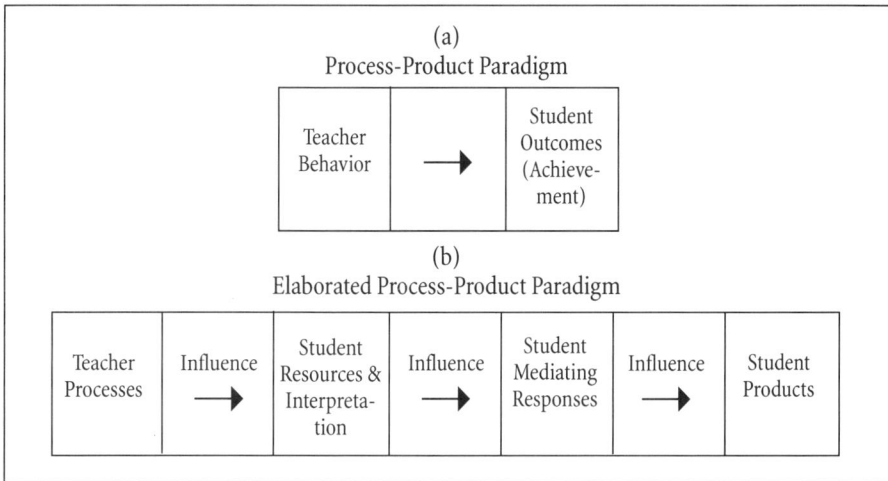

Figure 3. Research designs investigating effective instruction.

that predict or cause products (usually student achievement outcomes). Although useful in a descriptive sense, the basic process-product paradigm has been criticized as too restrictive because there is no accounting for events that intervene between teacher behaviors and student outcomes (Doyle, 1978). The consequences of this restricted view are limited findings that result in low correlations and methodological disputes. Additional criticisms of the basic process-product paradigm surround its inherent assumptions about causation (i.e., teachers cause student achievement), its formulation of rules of pedagogy without a normative base, and its emphasis on teacher behavior over the content being taught (Garrison & Macmillan, 1984).

The findings from research using the basic process-product paradigm are often equivocal; the paradigm is basically correlational rather than experimental in nature. There is little active manipulation of variables as in true experimental designs, and the basic process-product paradigm might be better termed a quasi-experimental design (Cook & Campbell, 1979). As such, process-product research is closer in spirit to evaluation rather than research because of the limited control over extraneous variables (Cronbach, 1982).

To overcome these difficulties, two additional paradigms need to be included to expand the basic process-product paradigm (see Doyle, 1978). The first is termed a *mediating-process paradigm* that takes into account student responses and the psychological processes governing learning. The second is termed a *classroom-ecology paradigm* that focuses on relationships between environmental demands and responses occurring in this natural setting. The elaborated process-product paradigm is shown in Figure 3(b). The expanded paradigm possesses the advantage of transcending the single (and simple) comparison of X (i.e., teacher behavior) and Y (i.e., student outcomes) by permitting the simultaneous examination of a range of variables (e.g., degree of structure, allocation of academic time, teacher feedback) in a large sample of classrooms using a variety of instructional approaches. Such "impact evaluations" (Gersten & Hauser, 1984) capitalize on the natural variation in teaching procedures, curriculum content, and classroom organization to determine what makes instruction effective.

Recognition of the complex nature of special education and the variety of interactions that may influence efficacy has resulted in evaluation practices that emphasize formative procedures concerned with general program improvement over summative procedures concerned solely with the classification (i.e., good vs. poor) of static programs. To accommodate what is known about effective schooling and instruction, evaluation efforts should be based on information reflecting the available research findings. The following example represents the ways in which research findings can be incorporated into a series of questions that may be used to evaluate a special education program (Utah Special Education Consortium Evaluation Task Force, 1986):

*Special Education
Evaluation Questions*

1.0 Are students achieving appropriate outcomes?

1.1 Have appropriate student outcomes in academic, vocational/life skills and social/behavioral areas been identified?

1.2 Are *all* ongoing monitoring procedures focused on final program outcomes?

1.3 Are program change processes directed by student outcome data?

2.0 Are staff using effective pedagogy?

2.1 Are the major instructional and management procedures validated for the target population and the curriculum outcome?

2.2 Is there a high level of engaged time?

2.3 Is the total instructional time managed to ensure achievement of the projected outcomes?

2.4 Are instructional practices congruent with prescribed outcomes?

2.5 Is at least 50% of the instructional time committed to the acquisition of new skills?

2.6 Are daily prescriptive and intervention procedures incorporating prerequisite skills and curriculum sequencing?

2.7 Are teacher/learner interactions consistent with the research literature on praise and feedback?

3.0 Are identification and placement procedures facilitative of student growth and consistent with applicable regulations?

3.1 Do screening procedures identify the high-risk students?

3.2 Have interventions relevant to the presenting problems been implemented and results documented prior to referral for assessment for possible special education services?

3.3 Are assessment practices appropriate for the problem and facilitative of instruction?

3.4 Are team classification decisions consistent with available assessment data and applicable regulations?

3.5 Are IEP goals and objectives team decisions and consistent with assessed student needs?

3.6 Are special education interventions delivered in the least restrictive environment?

4.0 Are instructional program coordination practices effective?

4.1 Are program needs and strengths being assessed for determining priorities for program change?

4.2 Are staff development activities identified, implemented, and evaluated consistent with priorities?

4.3 Is there effective coordination of interventions across instructional environments?

4.4 Are the roles and responsibilities of all system elements defined and clearly communicated to all involved in the education of special students?

5.0 Are community communication and involvement practices effective?

5.1 Are effective procedures in place to allow parent and community comments, suggestions, and concerns to be voiced and responded to at the program level?

5.2 Are there effective procedures for communicating program activities and rationales to parents and community?

5.3 Have available community resources been identified and used effectively?

# Philosophical Perspectives on the Efficacy of Special Education

Although research endeavors in special education reveal a positive trend toward more dynamic designs, there are still unanswered questions about the best way to study special education: How should the instructional situation be viewed? Should we examine small elements or large units? The answers that have been provided reveal fundamental differences about the theoretical and philosophical foundations of special education.

Heshusius (1982) suggested that a foundation provided by a predominantly mechanistic (i.e., behavioral) approach reduces special education teaching and learning to a subordinate level of rules and instrumentation. The resulting measurement and quantification of instruction does not operate at levels that are either meaningful or worthwhile for the learning requirements of the special education student. Heshusius warned that mechanistic assumptions are too narrow and simplistic, and, although recognizing that no one model holds ultimate truth or reality, suggested that special education practitioners have been trying to do the impossible— "to force the innately unpredictable into the predictable, the unmeasurable into the measurable, and wholeness into fragmentation" (p. 12).

The basic problem with a mechanistic approach is the demand that teachers become primarily behavioral engineers or technicians, a transformation that promotes the reduction of complex reality into quantifiable triviality. Optimal intervention requires an understanding of "complexity in its own right and the relationship of the whole to its parts, rather than trying to understand complexity by fragmenting it and reducing it to small, statistically measurable units over which one thinks one has control" (Heshusius, 1986, p. 463). This view about the nature of special education teaching and learning did not go unchallenged (Ulman & Rosenberg, 1986), and mechanistic approaches were credited with being the primary agent for the efficient evaluation and modification of the complexity surrounding special education programs (Kimball & Heron, 1988; Nelson & Polsgrove, 1984). Such debate has not been restricted to special education but rather extends to all educational research as witnessed by debate about positivism (i.e., behaviorism) and its influence on education (see Phillips, 1983, and response by Eisner,

1983). The debate led to a critical examination of the nature of educational research with particular attention to its philosophical underpinnings (e.g., Garrison, 1986; Macmillan & Garrison, 1984).

The debate in special education continued with Poplin's (1988b) criticism of the reductionistic tendencies found in all special education models whether they are based on medical, process, behavioral, or cognitive perspectives, and then suggested that holistic principles should be the basis for instructional practice (Poplin, 1988a). Similarly, Iano (1986) suggested that the predominant natural science-technical model (i.e., mechanistic) has failed to capture the complexity of the teaching-learning process and has also created an artificial distinction between researchers and practitioners. Researchers tend to reduce classroom behavior to a series of controlled or observable variables that fail to capture classroom reality while teachers often view such variables as minor contributors to the teaching-learning process and hence have little confidence in the generalizability of research findings. Iano's view was followed by commentary (e.g., Carnine, 1987; Forness & Kavale, 1987; Lloyd, 1987) either criticizing, expanding, or clarifying specific points to which Iano (1987) then responded.

These debates have served to focus attention on model-based practice in special education (Rosenberg & Jackson, 1988). Presently, the validity and worth of any particular special education model is practically impossible to determine. It may be the case that we need to accept the fact that multiple models may be equally productive for studying efficacy (Labouvie, 1975; Licht & Torgesen, 1989). Although different models may lead to different interpretations of observed intervention effects, all would be retained for possible utilization in classroom situations. Nonetheless, this relativism, or belief that judgments concerning the adequacy of conflicting educational models cannot be made, has been challenged (Phillips, 1983). For example, Soltis (1984), while encouraging tolerance for all educational models within an "associated community," emphasized that open-mindedness must not be mistakenly viewed as synonymous with empty-mindedness; special education professionals must exercise judgment when evaluating the efficacy of their interventions. Donmoyer (1985) asserted that relativism has contributed to special education being a solipsistic morass where any conclusion regarding the effectiveness of a particular intervention could be judged as positive as any other intervention even when conflicting findings exist about their efficacy.

Nevertheless, Rosenberg and Jackson (1988) discussed two issues that are of central importance in making intervention decisions. Both issues are predicated on the assumptions "that (a) changing the behaviors of students is a useful and appropriate educational goal, (b) the behavior changes are the product of specifiable activities that can be employed in other situations with the same or other students, and (c) changes are significant in the practical sense and are enduring either for the specific learners or for other populations of learners" (p. 30).

The first issue surrounds *instructional validity*, the degree to which a special education model can be relied upon to effect a certain outcome. The two important considerations are internal validity and external validity (Campbell

& Stanley, 1966; Cook & Campbell, 1979); internal validity refers to whether or not the intervention in question was responsible for observed behavior changes while external validity refers to the question of the generalizability of observed effects. From a mechanistic view, variables that might be considered "contaminating" (and thus may limit internal validity) would be viewed as important determinants of change and studied in their own right from a holistic perspective to insure external validity. Depending on your theoretical view, threats may not really be threats but rather the independent variables producing change. Thus, to insure a comprehensive perspective, instructional validity should not emphasize either internal or external validity but rather the nature of the independent variables and specific learning outcomes.

The second issue surrounds *outcome validity* and refers to the value of intervention activities in terms of the results being shown to possess educational importance (Howe, 1985). Outcome validity thus transcends philosophical perspectives by investigating the social utility of the intervention; whether it possesses functional relevance and contributes to meeting explicit goals and objectives for a particular special education student. For an applied field like special education, the evaluation of social utility should be integral to any assessment of intervention efficacy because it also addresses the question of accountability. Thus, a broader view of efficacy is achieved that encompasses the entire process of special education.

# Conclusion

Although research about effective schooling and instruction has produced an impressive set of findings, the generalizations have been far from prescriptive. For this reason, special education will remain a system that is variable, indeterminate, unpredictable, unlawful, and value-laden. As such, multiple special education models will need to be accepted because what works in one place may not work someplace else. Consequently, special education involves a degree of "uncertainty" (Glass, 1979) and "risk" (Kaplan, 1964) brought about because any intervention may or may not work.

The recognition of uncertainty and risk, however, does not preclude rational instructional planning for special education students. What uncertainty and risk do is make the teacher the central character in the special education process. Success or failure in special education is often the result of uncontrolled (and sometimes unknown) factors; consequently, a teacher must command options rather than truths in an effort to minimize risk by providing a satisfactory solution under conditions of uncertainty. A satisfactory solution is best achieved when dogmatic beliefs are replaced by rational choices that are best gleaned from the research literature, and it is of paramount importance that teachers gain insight into what constitutes best practice. The goal is to narrow the gap between the state of the art (what researchers have demonstrated is possible) and the state of the practice (current ways of providing instruction). Smith and West (1986) posed a series of questions that teachers may use to determine if they are providing state-of-the-art practice.

1. Do you upgrade your services by actively seeking information on new developments in your field?

2. Do you provide daily interactions with nonhandicapped, same-age peers for your students?

3. Is the program, including learning materials, appropriate for the student's chronological age?

4. Do you provide individualized instruction that is tailored for each student's individual needs?

5. Do parents contribute to the design of individualized program plans?

6. Does your program provide a planned transition process for students moving from school to community?

7. Does your program utilize the services of outside consultants to provide technical assistance at least once yearly?

8. Do you consider your program to be comprehensive in meeting all your student's needs?

9. Do you measure program effectiveness in terms of changes in daily performance in instructional, social, residential, and vocational environments?

10. Do you enjoy a high level of interagency cooperation and coordination?

Although state-of-the-art knowledge is important, it requires interpretation to provide a state of practice. This interpretation to produce a state of practice is the responsibility of the individual teacher, and how well it is accomplished is the critical factor in determining the success or failure of special education. Although the research base underlying special education can be specified, it can only be specified so much, and then the practitioner's own wisdom and experience enter to complete the intricate concatenation of events involved in producing an optimal special education teaching-learning process.

The effectiveness of special education ultimately includes elements of both science and art. Science refers to the theoretical and empirical foundation defining the state of knowledge while art refers to interpretation provided to initiate actual practice. Gage (1978) argued that practical enterprises in the real world (e.g., special education) possess both scientific and artistic components and provided analogies with medicine and engineering, where the scientific basis is unquestioned but artistic elements also abound.

To practice medicine and engineering requires a knowledge of much science: concepts, or variables, and interrelations in the form of strong or weak laws, generalizations, or trends. But using science to achieve practical ends requires artistry—the artistry that enters into knowing when to follow the implications of the laws, generalizations, and trends, and especially, when not to, and how to combine two or more laws or trends in solving a problem. (p. 18)

The movement from the state of the art to the state of the practice has been termed the *is/ought* dichotomy (Phillips, 1980): Research findings take an *is* form (i.e., X is Y) while practical implications take an *ought* form (i.e., A ought to do B). The *ought* form thus requires translation of research findings, and this translation process has been aided significantly by recent research-based special education methods texts (e.g., Bos & Vaughn, 1994; Kameenui & Simmons, 1990; Mastropieri & Scruggs, 1994). Nevertheless, specific applications require the sagacity and perspicacity of the individual special education practitioner that should not be limited by any research-based over-specification of the teaching-learning process. Like doctors and engineers, special education practitioners will need to go beyond the scientific basis of their work. A special education student is quite likely to present problems where scientific generalizations, principles, and suppositions will not apply directly and must be mediated through the teacher's own creative rendering of best practice. Therefore, the creativity of the individual special education practitioner must not be stifled, because quality education for special education students will always be based on the artful application of science.

# REFERENCES

Abrami, P. C., Cohen, P. A., & d'Appolonia, S. (1988). Implementation problems in meta-analysis. *Review of Educational Research, 58,* 151–179.

Achinstein, P., & Barker, F. (1969). *The legacy of logical positivism.* Baltimore: Johns Hopkins University Press.

Adelman, H. S., & Compas, B. E. (1977). Stimulant drugs and learning problems. *Journal of Special Education, 11,* 377–416.

Alderman, M. K. (1990). Motivation for at-risk students. *Educational Leadership, 48,* 27–30.

Allen, V. L. (1976). The helping relationship and socialization of children: Some perspectives on tutoring. In V. L. Allen (Ed.), *Children as teachers: Theory and research on tutoring* (pp. 9–25). New York: Academic Press.

Aman, M. G. (1980). Psychotropic drugs and learning problems: A selective review. *Journal of Learning Disabilities, 13,* 89–97.

American Academy of Pediatrics Committee on Drugs. (1970). An examination of the pharmacologic approach to learning impediments. *Pediatrics, 46,* 142–144.

American Academy of Pediatrics Council on Child Health. (1975). Medication for hyperkinetic children. *Pediatrics, 55,* 560–562.

Andreski, S. (1972). *Social sciences as sorcery.* London: Andre Deutsch.

Arena, J. I. (Ed.). (1969). *Teaching through sensory-motor experiences.* San Rafael, CA: Academic Therapy Publications.

Arter, J. A., & Jenkins, J. R. (1977). Examining the benefits and prevalence of modality considerations in special education. *Journal of Special Education, 11,* 281–298.

Arter, J. A., & Jenkins, J. R. (1979). Differential diagnosis-prescriptive teaching: A critical appraisal. *Review of Educational Research, 49,* 517–555.

Asarnow, J. R. (1992). Psychosocial intervention strategies for the depressed child: Approaches to treatment and prevention. *Child and Adolescent Psychiatric Clinics of North America, 1,* 257–283.

Asher, S. R., & Taylor, A. R. (1983). Social skills training with children: Evaluating processes and outcomes. *Studies in Educational Evaluation, 8,* 237–245.

Atkinson, R. C. (1975). Mnemotechnics in second-language learning. *American Psychologist, 30,* 821–828.

Baker, J. M., & Zigmond, N. (1990). Are regular education classes equipped to accommodate students with learning disabilities? *Exceptional Children, 56,* 515–526.

Balow, B. (1971). Percepual-motor activities in the treatment of severe reading disability. *Reading Teacher, 25,* 513–525.

Balow, B., & Brinkerhoff, R. (1983). Influences on special education evaluation. In R. O. Brinkerhoff, D. Brethower, T. Hluchjy, & J. Nowakowski (Eds.), *Program evaluation: A practitioner's guide for trainers and educators* (pp. xxiii–xxvii). Boston: Kluer-Nijoff.

Bangert-Downs, R. L. (1986). Review of developments in meta-analytic method. *Psychological Bulletin, 99,* 388–399.

Barbe, W. B., & Milone, M. N. (1981). What we know about modality strengths. *Educational Leadership, 38,* 378–380.

Barber, T. X. (1976). *Pitfalls in human research: Ten pivotal points.* New York: Pergamon Press.

Barkley, R. A. (1977). A review of stimulant drug research with hyperactive children. *Journal of Child Psychology and Psychiatry, 18,* 137–165.

Barkley, R. A. (1990). *Attention deficit hyperactivity disorder: A handbook for diagnosis and treatment.* New York: Guilford Press.

Barkley, R. A., & Cunningham, C. E. (1978). Do stimulant drugs improve the academic performance of hyperactive children? *Clinical Pediatrics, 17,* 85–92.

Barsch, R. H. (1967*). Achieving perceptual–motor efficiency: A space-oriented approach to learning.* Seattle, WA: Special Child Publications.

Baumeister, A. A. (1967). Learning abilities of the mentally retarded. In A. A. Baumeister (Ed.), *Mental retardation: Appraisal, education, and rehabilitation* (pp. 181–211). Chicago: Aldine Press.

Baumeister, A. A., & Kellas, G. (1971). Process variables in the paired associate learning of retardates. In N. R. Ellis (Ed.), *International review of research in mental retardation* (Vol. 5, pp. 221–270). New York: Academic Press.

Baumeister, A. A., Kupstas, F., & Klindworth, L. M. (1990). New morbidity: Implications for prevention of children's disabilities. *Exceptionality, 1,* 1–16.

Bay, M. R. (1985). Measuring the social position of the mainstreamed handicapped child. *Exceptional Children, 52,* 57–62.

Berk, R. A. (1984). An evaluation of procedures for computing an ability-achievement discrepancy score. *Journal of Learning Disabilities, 17,* 262–266.

Berkson, G., & Landesman-Dwyer, S. (1977). Behavioral research on severe and profound mental retardation. *American Journal of Mental Deficiency, 81,* 428–454.

Bickel, W. E., & Bickel, D. D. (1986). Effective schools, classrooms, and instruction: Implications for special education. *Exceptional Children, 52,* 489–500.

Blackorby, J., & Wagner, M. (1996). Longitudinal postschool outcomes of youth with disabilities: Findings from the National Longitudinal Study. *Exceptional Children, 62,* 399–414.

Blagg, N. (1991). *Can we teach intelligence? A comprehensive evaluation of Feuerstein's instrumental enrichment program.* Hillsdale, NJ: Erlbaum.

Borkowski, J. G., & Wanschura, P. B. (1974). Mediational processes in the retarded. In N. R. Ellis (Ed.), *International review of research in mental retardation* (Vol. 7, pp. 1–54). New York: Academic Press.

Bos, C. S., & Vaughn, S. (1994). *Strategies for teaching students with learning and behavior problems* (3rd ed.). Boston: Allyn & Bacon.

Bray, N. W. (1979). Strategy production in the retarded. In N. R. Ellis (Ed.), *Handbook of mental deficiency: Psychological theory and research* (2nd ed., pp. 699–726). Hillsdale, NJ: Erlbaum.

Bregman, J. D. (1991). Current developments in the understanding of mental retardation, Part II: Psychopathology. *Journal of American Academy of Child and Adolescent Psychiatry, 30,* 861–872.

Bregman, J. D., & Hodapp, R. M. (1991). Current developments in the understanding of mental retardation, Part I: Biological and phenomenological perspectives. *Journal of American Academy of Child and Adolescent Psychiatry, 30,* 707–719.

Brodbeck, M. (1962). Explanation, prediction, and "imperfect" knowledge. In H. Feigl & G. Maxwell (Eds.), *Minnesota studies in the philosophy of science, Vol. III.* Minneapolis: University of Minnesota Press.

Brooks, P. H., & Baumeister, A. A. (1977). A plea for consideration of ecological validity in the experimental psychology of mental retardation: A guest editorial. *American Journal of Mental Deficiency, 81,* 407–416.

Brooks, P. H., Sperber, R., & McCauley, C. (Eds.). (1984). *Learning and cognition in the mentally retarded.* Hillsdale, NJ: Erlbaum.

Brophy, J. E. (1982). How teachers influence what is taught and learned in classrooms. *Elementary School Journal, 83,* 1–13.

Brophy, J. E., & Good, T. L. (1986). Teacher behavior and student achievement. In M. C. Wittrock (Ed.), *Handbook of research on teaching* (3rd ed., pp. 328–375). New York: Macmillan.

Brown, A. L. (1974). The role of strategic behavior in retardate memory. In N. R. Ellis (Ed.), *International review of research in mental retardation* (Vol. 7, pp. 55–111). New York: Academic Press.

Bryan, T. (1991). Social problems and learning disabilities. In B. Y. L. Wong (Ed.), *Learning about learning disabilities* (pp. 195–229). San Diego: Academic Press.

Budoff, M., Thormann, M. J., & Gras, A. (1984). *Microcomputers in special education: An introduction to instructional applications.* Cambridge, MA: Brookline.

Burstein, L., & Guiton, G. W. (1984). Methodological perspectives on documenting program impact. In B. K. Keogh (Ed.), *Advances in special education* (Vol. 4, pp. 21–42). Greenwich, CT: JAI Press.

Bush, W. J., & Giles, M. T. (1977). *Aids to psycholinguistic teaching* (2nd ed.). Columbus, OH: Charles E. Merrill.

Cameron, J., & Pierce, W. D. (1994). Reinforcement, reward, and intrinsic motivation: A meta-analysis. *Review of Educational Research, 64,* 363–423.

Campbell, D. T. (1969). Reforms as experiments. *American Psychologist, 24,* 409–429.

Campbell, D. T., & Stanley, J. C. (1966). *Experimental and quasi-experimental designs for research.* Chicago: Rand McNally.

Campbell, M. (1975a). Pharmacotherapy in early infantile autism. *Biological Psychiatry, 10,* 399–423.

Campbell, M. (1975b). Psychopharmacology in childhood psychosis. *International Journal of Mental Health, 4,* 238–254.

Campbell, P., & Siperstein, G. M. (1994). *Improving social competence: A resource for elementary school teachers.* Boston: Allyn & Bacon.

Cantwell, D. P., & Carlson, G. A. (1978). Stimulants. In J. S. Werry (Ed.), *Pediatric psychopharmacology: The use of behavior modifying drugs in children* (pp. 171–207). New York: Brunner/Mazel.

Carbo, M. (1983). Research in reading and learning style: Implications for exceptional children. *Exceptional Children, 49,* 486–494.

Carbo, M. (1992). Giving unequal learners an equal chance: A reply to a biased critique of learning styles. *Remedial and Special Education, 13,* 19–29.

Carlberg, C., & Kavale, K. (1980). The efficacy of special versus regular class placement for exceptional children: A meta-analysis. *Journal of Special Education, 14,* 295–309.

Carlson, G. A., & Rapport, M. D. (1989). Diagnostic classification issues in attention-deficit hyperactivity disorder. *Psychiatric Annals, 19,* 576–583.

Carnine, D. (1987). A response to "False standards, a distorting and disintegrating effect on education, turning away from useful purposes, being inevitably unfulfilled, and remaining unrealistic and irrelevant." *Remedial and Special Education, 8*(1), 42–43.

Cartledge, G., Stupay, D., & Kaczala, C. (1986). Social skills and social perception of LD and nonhandicapped elementary-school students. *Learning Disability Quarterly, 9,* 226–234.

Carver, R. P. (1978). The case against statistical significance testing. *Harvard Educational Review, 48,* 378–399.

Casto, G., & Mastropieri, M. A. (1986). The efficacy of early intervention programs: A meta-analysis. *Exceptional Children, 52,* 417–424.

Cegelka, W. J., & Tyler, J. L. (1970). The efficacy of special class placement for the mentally retarded in proper perspective. *Training School Bulletin, 67,* 33–68.

Chaikind, S., Danielson, L. C., & Brauen, M. L. (1993). What do we know about the costs of special education? A selected review. *Journal of Special Education, 26,* 344–370.

Chapman, J. W. (1988). Learning disabled children's self-concepts. *Review of Educational Research, 58,* 347–371.

Christenson, S. L., Ysseldyke, J. E., & Thurlow, M. L. (1989). Critical instructional factors for students with mild handicaps: An integrative review. *Remedial and Special Education, 10,* 21–31.

Christopolos, F., & Renz, P. (1969). A critical examination of special education programs. *Journal of Special Education, 3,* 371–379.

Cohen, H. J., Birch, H. G., & Taft, L. T. (1970). Some considerations for evaluating the Doman-Delacato "patterning" method. *Pediatrics, 45,* 302–314.

Cohen, J. (1988). *Statistical power analysis for the behavioral sciences* (2nd ed.). Hillsdale, NJ: Erlbaum.

Cohen, P. A., Kulik, J. A., & Kulik, C. C. (1982). Educational outcomes of tutoring: A meta-analysis of findings. *American Educational Research Journal, 19,* 237–248.

Cohen, R. L. (1983). Individual differences in short-term memory. In N. R. Ellis (Ed.), *International review of research in mental retardation* (Vol. 11, pp. 43–77). New York: Academic Press.

Cohen, S. A. (1987). Instructional alignment: Searching for the magic bullet. *Educational Researcher, 16,* 16–20.

Combrinck-Graham, L. (1987). Commentary on drug treatment for behavioral control. *Clinical Pediatrics, 26,* 262–263.

Conduct Problems Prevention Research Group. (1992). A developmental and clinical model for the prevention of conduct disorder: The FAST Track Program. *Development and Psychopathology, 4,* 509–527.

Conners, C. K. (1973). Rating scales for use in drug studies with children (Special Issue: Pharmacology of Children). *Psychopharmacology Bulletin, 8,* 24–84.

Connors, C. K. (1980). *Food additives and hyperactive children.* New York: Plenum.

Conners, C. K., & Werry, J. S. (1979). Pharmacotherapy. In H. Quay & J. Werry (Eds.), *Psychopathological disorders of childhood* (2nd ed., pp. 336–386). New York: Wiley.

Cook, S. B., Scruggs, T. E., Mastropieri, M. A., & Casto, G. C. (1985–86). Handicapped students as tutors. *Journal of Special Education, 19,* 483–492.

Cook, T. D., & Campbell, D. T. (1979). *Quasi-experimentation: Design and analysis for field settings.* Chicago: Rand McNally.

Cooper, H., & Hedges, L. V. (Eds.). (1993). *The handbook of research synthesis.* New York: Russell Sage Foundation.

Cosden, M. M., & Abernathy, T. V. (1990). Microcomputer use in the schools: Teacher roles and instructional options. *Remedial and Special Education, 11,* 31–38.

Council for Learning Disabilities. (1986). Measurement and training of perceptual and perceptual-motor functions: A position statement. *Learning Disability Quarterly, 9,* 247.

Cowart, V. S. (1988). The ritalin controversy: What's made this drug's opponents hyperactive? *Journal of the American Medical Association, 259,* 2521–2523.

Cratty, B. (1969). *Perceptual-motor behavior and educational processes.* Springfield, IL: Charles C Thomas.

Crenshaw, T. M. (1997). *Attention deficit hyperactivity disorder and the efficacy of stimulant medication: A meta-analysis.* Unpublished doctoral dissertation, University of Virginia, Charlottesville.

Cronbach, L. J. (1982). *Designing evaluations of educational and social programs.* San Francisco: Jossey-Bass.

Cronbach, L. J., & Snow, R. E. (1977). *Aptitudes and instructional methods: A handbook for research on interactions.* New York: Irvington.

Cronbach, L. J., & Suppes, P. (1969). *Research for tomorrow's schools: Disciplined inquiry for education.* New York: Macmillan.

Delacato, C. H. (1959). *The treatment and prevention of reading problems: The neurological approach.* Springfield, IL: Charles C Thomas.

Delacato, C. H. (1966). *Neurological organization and reading.* Springfield, IL: Charles C Thomas.

Delquadri, J., Greenwood, C. R., Whorton, D., Carta, J. J., & Hall, R. V. (1986). Classwide peer tutoring. *Exceptional Children, 52,* 535–542.

Denham, C., & Lieberman, A. (Ed.). (1980). *Time to learn.* Washington, DC: National Institute of Education.

Denny, M. R. (1964). Research in learning and performance. In H. Stevens & R. Heber (Eds.), *Mental retardation: A review of research* (pp. 100–142). Chicago: University of Chicago Press.

Denny, M. R. (1966). A theoretical analysis and its application to training and the mentally retarded. In N. R. Ellis (Ed.), *International review of research in mental retardation* (Vol. 2, pp. 1–27). New York: Academic Press.

Deno, E. (1970). Special education as developmental capital. *Exceptional Children, 37,* 229–237.

Deno, E. (1973). *Instructional alternatives for exceptional children.* Reston, VA: Council for Exceptional Children.

Deno, S., Maruyama, G., Espin, C., & Cohen, C. (1990). Educating students with mild disabilities in general education classrooms: Minnesota alternatives. *Exceptional Children, 57,* 150–161.

Donmoyer, R. (1985). The rescue from relativism: Two failed attempts and an alternative strategy. *Educational Researcher, 14,* 13–20.

Doyle, W. (1978). Paradigms for research on teacher effectiveness. In L. S. Shulman (Ed.), *Review of research in education, 5,* 163–197.

Dudley-Marling, C. C., & Edmiaston, R. (1985). Social status of learning disabled children and adolescents: A review. *Learning Disability Quarterly, 8,* 189–204.

Dunkin, M. J., & Biddle, B. J. (1974). *The study of teaching.* New York: Holt, Rinehart & Winston.

Dunn, L. M. (1968). Special education for the mildly retarded—Is much of it justifiable? *Exceptional Children, 35,* 5–22.

Dunn, L. M., & Smith, J. O. (1967). *Peabody language development kits.* Circle Pines, MN: American Guidance Service.

Dunn, R. S. (1979). Learning—A matter of style. *Educational Leadership, 36,* 430–432.

Dunn, R. S. (1990). Bias over substance: A critical analysis of Kavale and Forness' report on modality-based instruction. *Exceptional Children, 56,* 352–356.

Dunn, R. S., & Dunn, K. J. (1978). *Teaching students through their individual learning styles.* Englewood Cliffs, NJ: Prentice-Hall.

Dunn, R. S., Dunn, K. J., & Price, G. E. (1979). *Learning style inventory.* Lawrence, KS: Price Systems.

DuPaul, G. J., & Stoner, G. (1994). *ADHD in the schools: Assessment and intervention strategies.* New York: Guilford Press.

Durlak, J. A., Fuhrman, T., & Lampman, C. (1991). Effectiveness of cognitive-behavior therapy for maladapting children: A meta-analysis. *Psychological Bulletin, 110,* 204–210.

Dush, D. M., Hirt, M. L., & Schroeder, H. E. (1989). Self-statement modification in the treatment of child behavior disorders: A meta-analysis. *Psychological Bulletin, 106,* 97–106.

Eisenberg, N. (1991). Meta-analytic contributions to the literature on prosocial behavior. *Personality and Social Psychology Bulletin, 17,* 273–282.

Eisner, E. (1979). *The educational imagination.* New York: Macmillan.

Eisner, E. W. (1983). Anastasia might still be alive, but the monarchy is dead. *Educational Researcher, 12,* 13–24.

Elliott, S. N., & Gresham, E. M. (1991). *Social skills intervention guide.* Circle Pines, MN: American Guidance Service.

Ellis, E. S., Lenz, B. K., & Sabornie, E. J. (1987). Generalization and adaptation of learning strategies to natural environments: Part I: Critical agents. *Remedial and Special Education, 8,* 6–20.

Ellis, N. R. (1963). The stimulus trace and behavioral inadequacy. In N. R. Ellis (Ed.), *Handbook of mental deficiency: Psychological theory and research* (pp. 134–158). New York: McGraw-Hill.

Ellis, N. R. (1970). Memory processes in retardates and normals. In N. R. Ellis (Ed.), *International review of research in mental retardation* (Vol. 4, pp. 1–32). New York: Academic Press.

Engelmann, S., Becker, W. C., Hanner, S., & Johnson, G. (1988). *Corrective reading program: Series guide* (rev. ed.). Chicago: Science Research Associates.

Engelmann, S., & Bruner, E. C. (1988). *Reading mastery: DISTAR reading.* Chicago: Science Research Associates.

Engelmann, S., & Carnine, D. W. (1982). *Theory of instruction: Principles and applications.* New York: Irvington.

Englert, C. S. (1983). Measuring special education teacher effectiveness. *Exceptional Children, 50,* 247–254.

Englert, C. S. (1984). Effective direct instruction practices in special education settings. *Remedial and Special Education, 5,* 38–47.

Englert, C. S., Tarrant, K. L., & Mariage, T. V. (1992). Defining and redefining instructional practice in special education: Perspectives on good teaching. *Teacher Education and Special Education, 15,* 62–87.

Epps, S., & Tindal, G. (1988). The effectiveness of differential programming in serving mildly handicapped students: Placement options and instructional programming. In M. Wang, M. Reynolds, & H. Walberg (Eds.), *Handbook of special education: Research and practice* (Vol. 2, pp. 172–215). Oxford: Pergamon Press.

Evans, R. A., & Bilsky, L. H. (1979). Clustering and categorical list retention in the mentally retarded. In N. R. Ellis (Ed.), *Handbook of mental deficiency: Psychological theory and research* (2nd ed., pp. 533–568). New York: McGraw-Hill.

Feingold, B. F. (1975). *Why your child is hyperactive.* New York: Random House.

Feingold, B. F. (1976). Hyperkinesis and learning disabilities linked to the ingestion of artificial food colors and flavors. *Journal of Learning Disabilities, 9,* 551–559.

Feingold, B. F., & Feingold, H. S. (1979). *The Feingold cookbook for hyperactive children.* New York: Random House.

Fish, B. (1960). Drug therapy in child psychiatry: Pharmacological aspects. *Comprehensive Psychiatry, 1,* 212–227.

Fisher, C. W., & Berliner, D. C. (1985). *Perspectives on instructional time.* White Plains, NY: Longman.

Fisher, M. A., & Zeaman, D. (1973). An attention-retention theory of retardate discrimination learning. In N. R. Ellis (Ed.), *International review of research in mental retardation* (Vol. 6, pp. 169–256). New York: Academic Press.

Fisher, R. A. (1956). *Statistical methods and scientific inference.* New York: Hafner.

Food color link to hyperactivity debated. (1980). *Pediatric New, 14,* 2.

Footlik, S. W. (1971). Perceptual-motor training and cognitive achievement: A survey of the literature. *Journal of Learning Disabilities, 3,* 40–49.

Forness, S. (1981). Concepts of school learning and behavior disorders: Implications for research and practice. *Exceptional Children, 48,* 56–64.

Forness, S. R. (1990). Summary of symposium on epidemiology: Educational aspects of epidemiology. *Academy on Mental Retardation Newsletter, 10*(2), 9–11.

Forness, S. R., & Kavale, K. (1984). Education of the mentally retarded: A note on policy. *Education and Training of the Mentally Retarded, 19,* 239–245.

Forness, S. R., & Kavale, K. A. (1987). Holistic inquiry and the scientific challenge in special education: A reply to Iano. *Remedial and Special Education, 8*(1), 47–51.

Forness, S. R., & Kavale, K. A. (1988). Psychopharmacologic treatment: A note on classroom effects. *Journal of Learning Disabilities, 21,* 144–147.

Forness, S. R., & Kavale, K. A. (1991). Social skill deficits as a primary learning disability: A note on problems with the ICLD diagnostic criteria. *Learning Disabilities Research and Practice, 6,* 44–49.

Forness, S. R., & Kavale, K. A. (1994). The Balkanization of special education: Proliferation of categories for new behavioral disorders. *Education and Treatment of Children, 17,* 215–217.

Forness, S. R., & Kavale, K. A. (1996a). Syndromes on the margins of mental retardation: Dual diagnosis and Balkanization. In A. Hilton (Ed.), *Promising practices in mental retardation and developmental disabilities* (pp. 59–73). Reston, VA: Council for Exceptional Children.

Forness, S. R., & Kavale, K. A. (1996b). Treating social skill deficits in children with learning disabilities: A meta-analysis of the research. *Learning Disability Quarterly, 19,* 2–13.

Forness, S. R., Kavale, K. A., Blum, I. M., & Lloyd, J. W. (1997). Mega-analysis of meta-analyses: What works in special education and related services. *Teaching Exceptional Children, 29,* 4–9.

Forness, S. R., & Knitzer, J. (1992). A new proposed definition and terminology to replace "Serious Emotional Disturbance" in the Individuals with Disabilities Education Act. *School Psychology Review, 21,* 12–20.

Frankenberger, W., Lozar, B., & Dallas, P. (1990). The use of stimulant medication to treat attention deficit hyperactive disorder (ADHD) in elementary school children. *Developmental Disabilities Bulletin, 18,* 1–13.

Friend, J., & McNutt, G. (1984). Resource room programs: Where are we now? *Exceptional Children, 51,* 150–155.

Frostig, M., & Horne, D. (1964). *The Frostig program for the development of visual perception.* Chicago: Follett.

Fuchs, D., & Fuchs, L. S. (1994). Inclusive schools movement and the radicalization of special education reform. *Exceptional Children, 60,* 294–309.

Fuchs, D., & Fuchs, L. S. (1995a). Special education can work. In J. M. Kauffman, J. W. Lloyd, D. P. Hallahan, & T. A. Astuto (Eds.), *Issues in educational placement: Students with emotional and behavior disorders* (pp. 363–377). Hillsdale, NJ: Erlbaum.

Fuchs, D., & Fuchs, L. S. (1995b). What's "special" about special education? *Phi Delta Kappan, 76,* 22–30.

Fuchs, L. S., & Fuchs, D. (1986). Effects of systematic formative evaluation: A meta-analysis. *Exceptional Children, 53,* 199–208.

Fuchs, L. S., Fuchs, D., & Bishop, N. (1992). Teacher planning for students with learning disabilities: Differences between general and special educators. *Learning Disabilities Research and Practice, 7,* 120–128.

Fuchs, L. S., Fuchs, D., & Deno, S. L. (1985). The importance of goal ambitiousness and goal mastery to student achievement. *Exceptional Children, 52,* 63–71.

Gadow, K. D. (1983). Effects of stimulant drugs on academic performance in hyperactive and learning disabled children. *Journal of Learning Disabilities, 16,* 290–299.

Gage, N. L. (1978). *The scientific basis of the art of teaching.* New York: Teachers College Press, Columbia University.

Garber, H. L. (1988). *The Milwaukee Project: Preventing mental retardation in children at risk.* Washington, DC: American Association on Mental Retardation.

Garrison, J. W. (1986). Some principles of postpositivistic philosophy of science. *Educational Researcher, 15,* 12–18.

Garrison, J. W., & Macmillan, C. J. B. (1984). A philosophical critique of process-product research on teaching. *Educational Theory, 34,* 255–274.

Gartner, A., & Lipsky, D. K. (1987). Beyond special education: Toward a quality system for all students. *Harvard Educational Review, 57,* 367–395.

Gergen, K. J. (1973). Social psychology as history. *Journal of Personality and Social Psychology, 26,* 309–320.

Gersten, R., Carnine, D., & Woodward, J. (1987). Direct instruction research: The third decade. *Remedial and Special Education, 8,* 48–56.

Gersten, R., & Hauser, C. (1984). The case for impact evaluations in special education. *Remedial and Special Education, 5,* 16–24.

Gersten, R., & Keating, T. (1987). Long-term benefits from direct instruction. *Educational Leadership, 44,* 28–31.

Gersten, R., Woodward, J., & Darch, C. (1986). Direct instruction: A research-based approach to curriculum design and teaching. *Exceptional Children, 53,* 17–31.

Getman, G. N. (1965). The visuomotor complex in the acquisition of learning skills. In J. Hellmuth (Ed.), *Learning disorders* (Vol. 1, pp. 49–76). Seattle, WA: Special Child Publications.

Gettinger, M. B. (1991). Learning time and retention differences between non-disabled students and students with learning disabilities. *Learning Disability Quarterly, 14,* 179–189.

Gillingham, A., & Stillman, B. (1968). *Remedial teaching for children with specific disability in reading, spelling, and penmanship.* Cambridge, MA: Educator's Publishing Service.

Gittelman, R., & Kanner, A. (1986). Psychopharmacology. In H. Quay & J. Werry (Eds.), *Psychopathological disorders of childhood* (3rd ed.). New York: John Wiley.

Glass, G. V. (1976). Primary, secondary, and meta-analysis of research. *Educational Researcher, 5,* 3–8.

Glass, G. V. (1977). Integrating findings: The meta-analysis of research. In L. S. Shulman (Ed.), *Review of research in education, 5,* 351–379.

Glass, G. V. (1979). Policy for the unpredictable (uncertainty research and policy). *Educational Researcher, 8,* 12–14.

Glass, G. V., McGaw, B., & Smith, M. L. (1981). *Meta-analysis in social research.* Beverly Hills, CA: Sage.

Glass, G. V., & Robbins, M. P. (1967). A critique of experiments on the role of neurological organization in reading performance. *Reading Research Quarterly, 3,* 5–51.

Glass, G. V., & Smith, M. L. (1979). Meta-analysis of research on class size and achievement. *Educational Evaluation and Policy Analysis, 1,* 2–16.

Goldman, S. R., & Pellegrino, J. W. (1987). Information processing and educational microcomputer technology: Where do we go from here? *Journal of Learning Disabilities, 20,* 144–154.

Good, T. L. (1983). Classroom research: A decade of progress. *Educational Psychologist, 18,* 127–144.

Goodman, L. (1990). *Time and learning in the special education classroom.* Albany, NY: State University of New York Press.

Goodman, L., & Hammill, D. (1973). The effectiveness of the Kephart-Getman activities in developing perceptual-motor and cognitive skills. *Focus on Exceptional Children, 4,* 1–9.

Gottlieb, J., Alter, M., & Gottlieb, B. W. (1991). Mainstreaming academically handicapped children in urban schools. In J. W. Lloyd, N. N. Singh, & A. C. Repp (Eds.), *The regular education initiative: Alternative perspectives on concepts, issues, and models* (pp. 95–112). Sycamore, IL: Sycamore.

Gray, S., Ramsey, B., & Klaus, R. (1982). *From 3 to 20: The early training project.* Baltimore: University Park Press.

Greenwood, C. R. (1991). Longitudinal analysis of time, engagement, and achievement in at-risk versus non-risk students. *Exceptional Children, 57,* 521–534.

Greenwood, C. R., Carta, J. J., Hart, B., Kamps, D., Terry, D., Delquadri, J. C., Walker, D., & Risley, T. (1992). Out of the laboratory and into the community: Twenty-six years of applied behavior analysis at the Juniper Gardens Children's Center. *American Psychologist, 47,* 1464–1474.

Gresham, F. M. (1981). Social skills training with handicapped children: A review. *Review of Educational Research, 51,* 139–176.

Gresham, F. M. (1983). Social validity in the assessment of children's social competence: Establishing standards for social competency. *Journal of Psychoeducational Assessment, 1,* 297–307.

Gresham, F. M. (1986). Conceptual and definitional issues in the assessment of social skills: Implications for classification and training. *Journal of Clinical Child Psychology, 15,* 16–25.

Gresham, F. M. (1992). Social skills and learning disabilities: Causal, concomitant, or correlational? *School Psychology Review, 21,* 348–360.

Gresham, F. M., & Elliott, S. N. (1990). *Social skills rating system.* Circle Pines, MN: American Guidance Service.

Guevremont, D. C., & Dumas, M. C. (1994). Peer relationship problems and disruptive behavior disorders. *Journal of Emotional and Behavioral Disorders, 2,* 164–172.

Guskin, S. L., & Spicker, H. H. (1968). Educational research in mental retardation. In N. R. Ellis (Ed.), *International review of research in mental retardation* (Vol. 3, pp. 217–278). New York: Academic Press.

Haertel, G. D., Walberg, H. J., & Weinstein, T. (1983). Psychological models of educational performance: A theoretical synthesis of constructs. *Review of Educational Research, 53,* 75–92.

Hagin, R. A. (1973). Models of intervention with learning disabilities: Ephemeral and otherwise. *School Psychology Monograph, 1,* 1–24.

Hallahan, D. P., & Cruickshank, W. M. (1973). *Psychoeducational foundations of learning disabilities.* Englewood Cliffs, NJ: Prentice-Hall.

Hallahan, D. P., & Kauffman, J. M. (1977). Labels, categories, behaviors: ED, LD, and EMR reconsidered. *Journal of Special Education, 11,* 139–149.

Hallahan, D. P., & Kauffman, J. M. (1994). Toward a culture of diversity in the aftermath of Deno and Dunn. *Journal of Special Education, 27,* 496–508.

Hallahan, D. P., Keller, C. E., McKinney, J. D., Lloyd, J. W., & Bryan, T. (1988). Examining the research base of the regular education initiative: Efficacy studies and the adaptive learning environments model. *Journal of Learning Disabilities, 21,* 29–35.

Hallenbeck, B. A., & Kauffman, J. M. (1995). How does observational learning affect the behavior of students with emotional or behavioral disorders? A review of research. *Journal of Special Education, 29,* 45–71.

Hammill, D. D., Goodman, L., & Wiederholt, J. L. (1974). Visual-motor processes: Can we train them? *Reading Teacher, 27,* 469–478.

Hammill, D. D., & Larsen, S. C. (1974). The effectiveness of psycholinguistic training. *Exceptional Children, 41,* 5–14.

Hammill, D. D., & Larsen, S. C. (1978). The effectiveness of psycholinguistic training: A reaffirmation of position. *Exceptional Children, 44,* 402–414.

Hammill, D. D., & Wiederholt, J. L. (1972). *The resource room: Rationale and implementation.* Philadelphia: JSE Press.

Haynes, M. C., & Jenkins, J. R. (1986). Reading instruction in special education resource rooms. *American Educational Research Journal, 23,* 161–190.

Hazel, J. S., Schumaker, J. B., Sherman, J. A., & Sheldon-Wildgen, J. (1981). *ASSET: A social skills program for adolescents.* Champaign, IL: Research Press.

Hedges, L. V., & Olkin, I. (1985). *Statistical methods for meta-analysis.* New York: Academic Press.

Heller, K. A., Holtzman, W. H., & Messick, S. (1982). *Placing children in special education: A strategy for equity.* Washington, DC: National Academy Press.

Heshusius, L. (1982). At the heart of the advocacy dilemma: A mechanistic word view. *Exceptional Children, 49,* 6–13.

Heshusius, L. (1986). Paradigm shifts and special education: A response to Ulman and Rosenberg. *Exceptional Children, 52,* 461–465.

Hewett, F. M., & Forness, S. R. (1984). *Education of exceptional learners.* Newton, MA: Allyn & Bacon.

Howe, K. (1985). Two dogmas of educational research. *Educational Researcher, 14,* 10–18.

Hughes, J. N., & Sullivan, K. A. (1988). Outcome assessment in social skills training with children. *Journal of School Psychology, 26,* 167–183.

Hunter, J. E., Schmidt, F. L., & Jackson, G. B. (1982). *Meta-analysis: Cumulating research findings across studies.* Beverly Hills, CA: Sage.

Iano, R. P. (1986). The study and development of teaching: With implications for the advancement of special education. *Remedial and Special Education, 7*(5), 50–61.

Iano, R. P. (1987). Rebuttal: Neither the absolute certainty of prescriptive law nor a surrender to mysticism. *Remedial and Special Education, 8*(1), 52–61.

Itard, J. M. G. (1806/1962). *The wild boy of Aveyron.* (G. Humphrey & M. Humphrey, Trans.). New York: Appleton-Century-Crofts. (Original work published 1806.)

Jackson, G. B. (1980). Methods for integrative reviews. *Review of Educational Research, 50,* 438–460.

Jenkins, J. R., & Pany, D. (1978). Standardized achievement tests: How useful for special education? *Exceptional Children, 44,* 448–453.

Jensen, A. R. (1970). A theory of primary and secondary familial mental retardation. In N. R. Ellis (Ed.), *International review of research in mental retardation* (Vol. 4, pp. 33–106). New York: Academic Press.

Joyce, B., & Weil, M. (1972). *Models of teaching.* Englewood Cliffs, NJ: Prentice-Hall.

Kail, R. V., & Leonard, L. B. (1986). Sources of word-finding problems in language-impaired children. In S. J. Ceci (Ed.), *Handbook of cognitive, social, and neuropsychological aspects of learning disabilities* (Vol. 1, pp. 185–202). Hillsdale, NJ: Erlbaum.

Kameenui, E. J., & Simmons, D. C. (1990). *Designing instructional strategies: The prevention of academic learning problems.* Columbus, OH: Merrill.

Kaplan, A. (1964). *The conduct of inquiry.* San Francisco: Chandler.

Kauffman, J. M. (1981). Historical trends and contemporary issues in special education in the United States. In J. M. Kauffman & D. P. Hallahan (Eds.), *Handbook of special education* (pp. 3–23). Englewood Cliffs, NJ: Prentice-Hall.

Kauffman, J. M. (1993). How we might achieve the radical reform of special education. *Exceptional Children, 60,* 6–16.

Kauffman, J. M., & Hallahan, D. P. (Eds.). (1995). *The illusion of full inclusion: A comprehensive critique of a current special education bandwagon.* Austin, TX: PRO ED.

Kauffman, J. M., & Lloyd, J. W. (1995). A sense of place: The importance of placement issues in contemporary special education. In J. M. Kauffman, J. W. Lloyd, D. P. Hallahan, & T. A. Astuto (Eds.), *Issues in educational placement: Students with emotional and behavioral disorders* (pp. 3–19). Hillsdale, NJ: Erlbaum.

Kauffman, J. M., & Pullen, P. L. (1996). Eight myths about special education. *Focus on Exceptional Children, 28*(5), 1–12.

Kaufman, M. E., & Alberto, P. A. (1976). Research on efficacy of special education for the mentally retarded. In N. R. Ellis (Ed.), *International review of research in mental retardation* (Vol. 8, pp. 225–255). New York: Academic Press.

Kavale, K. A. (1979). Mainstreaming: The genesis of an idea. *The Exceptional Child, 26,* 3–21.

Kavale, K. A. (1981). Functions of the Illinois Test of Psycholinguistic Abilities (ITPA): Are they trainable? *Exceptional Children, 47,* 496–510.

Kavale, K. A. (1982a). The efficacy of stimulant drug treatment for hyperactivity: A meta-analysis. *Journal of Learning Disabilities, 15,* 280–289.

Kavale, K. A. (1982b). Psycholinguistic training programs: Are there differential treatment effects? *The Exceptional Child, 29,* 21–30.

Kavale, K. A. (1984). Potential advantages of the meta-analysis technique for research in special education. *Journal of Special Education, 18,* 61–72.

Kavale, K. A. (1987). Theoretical quandaries in learning disabilities. In S. Vaughn & C. Bos (Eds.), *Research in learning disabilities: Issues and future directions* (pp. 111–131). Boston: Little, Brown/College-Hill.

Kavale, K. A., & Forness, S. R. (1983). Hyperactivity and diet treatment: A meta-analysis of the Feingold hypothesis. *Journal of Learning Disabilities, 16,* 324–330.

Kavale, K. A., & Forness, S. R. (1987). Substance over style: Assessing the efficacy of modality testing and teaching. *Exceptional Children, 54,* 228–234.

Kavale, K. A., & Forness, S. R. (1990). Substance over style: A rejoinder to Dunn's animadversions. *Exceptional Children, 56,* 357–361.

Kavale, K. A., & Forness, S. R. (1992). Learning difficulties and memory problems in mental retardation: A meta-analysis of theoretical perspectives. In T. Scruggs & M. Mastropieri (Eds.), *Advances in learning and behavior* (Vol. 7, pp. 177–219). Greenwich, CT: JAI Press.

Kavale, K. A., & Forness, S. R. (1994). Models and theories: Their influence on research in learning disabilities. In S. Vaughn & C. Bos (Eds.), *Research issues in learning disabilities: Theory, methodology, assessment, and ethics* (pp. 38–65). New York: Springer-Verlag.

Kavale, K. A., & Forness, S. R. (1995). Social skill deficits and training: A meta-analysis of the research in learning disabilities. In T. E. Scruggs & M. A. Mastropieri (Eds.), *Advances in learning and behavioral disabilities* (Vol. 9, pp. 119–160). Greenwich, CT: JAI Press.

Kavale, K. A., & Forness, S. R. (1996). Defining emotional or behavioral disorders: Divergence and convergence. In T. E. Scruggs & M. A. Mastropieri (Eds.), *Advances in learning and behavioral disabilities* (Vol. 10A, pp. 1–45). Greenwich, CT: JAI Press.

Kavale, K. A., Mathur, S. R., Forness, S. R., Rutherford, R. B., & Quinn, M. M. (1997). Effectiveness of social skills training for students with behavior disorders: A meta-analysis. In T. E. Scruggs & M. A. Mastropieri (Eds.), *Advances in learning and behavioral disabilities* (Vol. 11, pp. 1–16). Greenwich, CT: JAI Press.

Kavale, K. A., & Mattson, P. D. (1983). One jumped off the balance beam: Meta-analysis of perceptual-motor training. *Journal of Learning Disabilities, 16,* 165–173.

Kavale, K. A., & Nye, C. (1984). The effectiveness of drug treatment for severe behavior disorders: A meta-analysis. *Behavioral Disorders, 9,* 117–130.

Kavale, K. A., & Reese, J. H. (1991). Teacher beliefs and perceptions about learning disabilities: A survey of Iowa practitioners. *Learning Disability Quarterly, 14,* 141–160.

Kennedy, C. H., & Shukla, S. (1995). Social interaction research for people with autism as a set of past, current, and emerging propositions. *Behavioral Disorders, 21,* 21–35.

Kephart, N. C. (1960). *The slow learner in the classroom.* Columbus, OH: Merrill.

Kephart, N. C. (1972). On the value of empirical data in learning disability. *Journal of Learning Disabilities, 4,* 393–395.

Kimball, W. H., & Heron, T. E. (1988). A behavioral commentary on Poplin's discussion of reductionistic fallacy and holistic/constructivist principles. *Journal of Learning Disabilities, 21,* 425–428.

King, B. H., State, M., Davanzo, P., Shah, B., & Dykens, E. (1997). Mental retardation: A review of the past 10 years (Part I). *Journal of the American Academy of Child and Adolescent Psychiatry, 36,* 1656–1663.

Kirk, S. A. (1958). *Early education of the mentally retarded: An experimental study.* Urbana: University of Illinois Press.

Kirk, S. A. (1964). Research in education. In H. A. Stevens & R. Heber (Eds.), *Mental retardation: A review of research.* Chicago: University of Chicago Press.

Kirk, S. A., & Kirk, W. D. (1971). *Psycholinguistic learning disabilities: Diagnosis and remediation.* Urbana: University of Illinois Press.

Kirk, S. A., McCarthy, J. J., & Kirk, W. D. (1968). *Illinois Test of Psycholinguistic Abilities* (rev. ed.). Urbana: University of Illinois Press.

Klein, D. F., Gittelman, R., Quitkin, F. M., & Rifkin, A. (1980). *Diagnosis and drug treatment of psychiatric disorders: Adults and children* (2nd ed.). Baltimore: Williams & Wilkins.

Kramer, J. J., Piersel, W. C., & Glover, J. A. (1988). Cognitive and social development of mildly retarded children. In C. Wang, C. Reynolds, & J. Walberg (Eds.), *Handbook of special education: Research and practice* (Vol. 2, pp. 43–58). New York: Pergamon Press.

Labouvie, E. W. (1975). The dialectical nature of measurement activities in the behavioral sciences. *Human Development, 18,* 205–222.

Ladd, G. W. (1984). Social skill training with children: Issues in research and practice. *Clinical Psychology Review, 4,* 317–337.

LaGreca, A. M. (1987). Children with learning disabilities: Interpersonal skills and social competence. *Journal of Reading, Writing, and Learning Disabilities International, 3,* 167–185.

LaGreca, A. M, & Vaughn, S. (1992). Social functioning of individuals with learning disabilities. *School Psychology Review, 21,* 340–347.

Larrivee, B. (1981). Modality preference as a model for differentiating beginning reading instruction: A review of the issues. *Learning Disability Quarterly, 4,* 180–188.

Larrivee, B. (1986). Effective teaching for mainstreamed students is effective teaching for all students. *Teacher Education and Special Education, 9,* 173–179.

Larsen, S. C., Parker, R. M., & Hammill, D. D. (1982). Effectiveness of psycholinguistic training: A response to Kavale. *Exceptional Children, 49,* 60–66.

Leinhardt, G., & Pallay, A. (1982). Restrictive educational settings: Exile or haven? *Review of Educational Research, 52,* 557–578.

Leinhardt, G., Zigmond, N., & Cooley, W. W. (1981). Reading instruction and its effects. *American Educational Research Journal, 18,* 343–361.

Levin, J. R. (1983). Pictorial strategies for school learning: Practical illustrations. In M. Pressley & J. R. Levin (Eds.), *Cognitive strategy research: Educational applications* (pp. 213–237). New York: Springer-Verlag.

Lew, F. (1977). The Feingold diet, experienced (letter). *Medical Journal of Australia, 1,* 190.

Lewis, R. B. (1993). *Special education technology: Classroom applications.* Pacific Grove, CA: Brookes.

Licht, B. G. (1983). Cognitive-motivational factors that contribute to the achievement of learning disabled children. *Journal of Learning Disabilities, 16,* 483–490.

Licht, B. G., & Torgesen, J. K. (1989). Natural science approaches to questions of subjectivity. *Journal of Learning Disabilities, 22,* 418–419.

Lieber, J., & Semmel, M. I. (1985). Effectiveness of computer application to instruction with mildly handicapped learners: A review. *Remedial and Special Education, 6,* 5–12.

Lindblom, C. E., & Cohen, D. K. (1979). *Usable knowledge: Social science and social problem solving.* New Haven, CT: Yale University Press.

Lipsky, D. K., & Gartner, A. (1989). *Beyond separate education: Quality education for all.* Baltimore: Brookes.

Lloyd, J. W. (1984). How shall we individualize instruction—Or should we? *Remedial and Special Education, 5*(1), 7–15.

Lloyd, J. W. (1987). The art and science of research on teaching. *Remedial and Special Education, 8*(1), 44–46.

Lovitt, T. C. (1984). *Tactics for teaching.* New York: Merrill/Macmillan.

Luckasson, R., Coulter, D., Polloway, E. A., Reiss, S., Schalock, R. L., Snell, M. E., Spitalnik, D. M., & Stark, J. A. (1992). *Mental retardation: Definition, classification, and systems of supports.* Washington, DC: American Association on Mental Retardation.

Lund, K. A., Foster, G. E., & McCall-Perez, G. C. (1978). The effectiveness of psycholinguistic training: A reevaluation. *Exceptional Children, 44,* 310–319.

Maag, J. W. (1989). Assessment in social skills training: Methodological and conceptual issues for research and practice. *Remedial and Special Education, 53,* 519–569.

Maag, J. W. (1993). Promoting social skills training in general education classrooms: Issues and tactics for collaborative consultation. *Monographs in Behavioral Disorders, 16,* 30–42.

Mackenzie, D. E. (1983). Research for school improvement: An appraisal of some recent trends. *Educational Researcher, 12*(4), 5–17.

Macmillan, C. J. B., & Garrison, J. W. (1984). Using the "new philosophy of science" in criticizing current research traditions in education. *Educational Researcher, 13,* 15–21.

MacMillan, D. L. (1971). Special education for the mildly retarded: Servant or savant? *Focus on Exceptional Children, 2,* 1–11.

MacMillan, D. L. (1989). Mild mental retardation: Emerging issues. In G. A. Robinson, J. R. Patton, E. A. Polloway, & L. R. Sargent (Eds.), *Best practices in mild mental disabilities* (pp. 1–20). Reston, VA: Council for Exceptional Children, Division on Mental Retardation.

MacMillan, D. L., & Forness, S. R. (1993). Mental retardation. In M. C. Alkin (Ed.), *Encyclopedia of education research* (pp. 825–830). New York: McGraw-Hill.

MacMillan, D. L., Gresham, F. M., & Forness, S. R. (1996). Full inclusion: An empirical perspective. *Behavioral Disorders, 21,* 145–159.

MacMillan, D. L., Gresham, F. M., & Siperstein, G. N. (1993). Conceptual and psychometric concerns about the 1992 AAMR definition of mental retardation. *American Journal on Mental Retardation, 98,* 325–335.

MacMillan, D. L., Gresham, F. M., & Siperstein, G. N. (1995). Heightened concerns over the 1992 AAMR definition: Advocacy versus precision. *American Journal on Mental Retardation, 100,* 87–97.

MacMillan, D. L., & Hendrick, I. G. (1993). Evolution and legacies. In J. I. Goodlad & T. C. Lovitt (Eds.), *Integrating general and special education* (pp. 23–48). Columbus, OH: Merrill/ Macmillan.

MacMillan, D. L., & Meyers, C. E. (1984). Molecular research and molar learning. In H. Brooks, R. Sperber, & C. McCauley (Eds.), *Learning and cognition in the mentally retarded* (pp. 473–492). Hillsdale, NJ: Erlbaum.

MacMillan, D. L., Siperstein, G. N., & Gresham, F. M. (1996). A challenge to the viability of mild mental retardation as a diagnostic category. *Exceptional Children, 62,* 356–371.

Maher, C. A., & Bennett, R. E. (1984). *Planning and evaluating special education services.* Englewood Cliffs, NJ: Prentice-Hall.

Malouf, D. B., Jamison, P. J., Kercher, M. H., & Carlucci, C. M. (1991). Integrating computer software into effective instruction. *Teaching Exceptional Children, 23,* 54–56.

Mann, L. (1970). Perceptual training: Misdirections and redirections. *American Journal of Orthopsychiatry, 40,* 30–38.

Mann, L. (1971a). Perceptual training revisited: The training of nothing at all. *Rehabilitation Literature, 32,* 322–327, 335.

Mann, L. (1971b). Psychometric phrenology and the new faculty psychology: The case against ability assessment and training. *Journal of Special Education, 5,* 3–14.

Mann, L. (1979). *On the trail of process.* New York: Grune & Stratton.

Mann, L., & Phillips, W. A. (1967). Fractional practices in special education: A critique. *Exceptional Children, 33,* 311–317.

Martin, C. J. (1978). Mediational processes in the retarded: Implications for teaching reading. In N. R. Ellis (Ed.), *International review of research in mental retardation* (Vol. 9, pp. 61–84). New York: Academic Press.

Martin, S. L., Ramey, C. T., & Ramey, S. L. (1990). The prevention of intellectual impairment in children of impoverished families: Findings of a randomized trial of educational daycare. *American Journal of Public Health, 80,* 844–847.

Mastropieri, M. A., & Scruggs, T. E. (1989). Constructing more meaningful relationships: Mnemonic instruction for special populations. *Educational Psychology Review, 1,* 83–111.

Mastropieri, M. A., & Scruggs, T. E. (1991). *Teaching students ways to remember: Strategies for learning mnemonically.* Cambridge, MA: Brookline Books.

Mastropieri, M. A., & Scruggs, T. E. (1994). *Effective instruction for special education* (2nd ed.). Austin, TX: PRO-ED.

Mastropieri, M. A., Scruggs, T. E., Bakken, J. P., & Whedon, C. (1996). Reading comprehension: A synthesis of research in learning disabilities. In T. E. Scruggs & M. A. Mastropieri (Eds.), *Advances in learning and behavioral disabilities* (Vol. 10, pp. 277–303). Greenwich, CT: JAI Press.

Mastropieri, M. A., Scruggs, T. E., & Fulk, B. J. (1990). Teaching abstract vocabulary to LD students with the keyword method: Effects on comprehension and recall. *Journal of Learning Disabilities, 23,* 92–107.

Mastropieri, M. A., Scruggs, T. E., Levin, J. R., Gaffney, J. S., & McLoone, B. B. (1985). Mnemonic vocabulary instruction for learning disabled students. *Learning Disability Quarterly, 8,* 57–63.

Mastropieri, M. A., Scruggs, T. E., Whittaker, M. E. S., & Bakken, J. P. (1994). Applications of mnemonic strategies with students with mental disabilities. *Remedial and Special Education, 15,* 34–43.

Mathur, S. R., & Rutherford, R. B. (1991). Peer-mediated interventions promoting social skills of children and youth with behavioral disorders. *Education and Treatment of Children, 14,* 227–242.

Mathur, S. R., & Rutherford, R. B. (1994). Success of social skills training with delinquent youth: Some critical issues. In T. E. Scruggs & M. A. Mastropieri (Eds.), *Advances in learning and behavioral disabilities* (Vol. 8, pp. 147–160). Hillsdale, NJ: Erlbaum.

Mattes, J. A. (1983). The Feingold diet: A current reappraisal. *Journal of Learning Disabilities, 16,* 319–323.

McGinnis, E., Goldstein, A., Sprafkin, R., & Gershaw, N. (1984). *Skill streaming the elementary school child: A guide for teaching prosocial skills.* Champaign, IL: Research Press.

McGrath, J. E., Martin, J., & Kulka, R. A. (1982). *Judgment calls in research.* Beverly Hills, CA: Sage.

McIntosh, R., Vaughn, S., & Zaragoza, N. (1991). A review of social interventions for students with learning disabilities. *Journal of Learning Disabilities, 24,* 451–458.

McLoughlin, J. A., & Kelly D. (1982). Issues facing the resource teacher. *Learning Disability Quarterly, 5,* 58–64.

Medley, D. M. (1982). Teacher effectiveness. In H. E. Mitzel (Ed.), *Encyclopedia of educational research* (5th ed., pp. 1894–1903). New York: Free Press.

Meyers, C. E., MacMillan, D. L., & Yoshida, R. K. (1980). Regular class education of EMR students, from efficacy to mainstreaming: A review of issues and research. In J. Gottlieb (Ed.), *Educating mentally retarded persons in the mainstream.* Baltimore: University Park Press.

Minskoff, E. (1975). Research on psycholinguistic training: Critique and guidelines. *Exceptional Children, 42,* 136–144.

Mitroff, I. I., & Featheringham, T. R. (1974). On systematic problem solving and the error of the third kind. *Behavioral Science, 19,* 383–393.

Morrison, D. E., & Henkel, R. E. (Eds.). (1970). *The significance test controversy: A reader.* Chicago: Aldine.

Morsink, C. V., Soar, R. S., Soar, R. M., & Thomas, R. (1986). Research on teaching: Opening the door to special education classrooms. *Exceptional Children, 53*(1), 32–40.

National Advisory Committee on Hyperkinesis and Food Additives. (1980). *Final report to the Nutrition Foundation.* New York: The Nutrition Foundation.

Nelson, C. M., & Polsgrove, L. (1984). Behavior analysis in special education; White rabbit or white elephant. *Remedial and Special Education, 5,* 6–15.

Newcomb, A. F., Bukowski, W. M., & Pattee, L. (1993). Children's peer relations: A meta-analytic review of popular, rejected, neglected, controversial, and average sociometric status. *Psychological Bulletin, 113,* 99–128.

Newcomer, P., Larsen, S., & Hammill, D. (1975). A response. *Exceptional Children, 42,* 144–148.

Niemic, R., Samson, G., Weinstein, T., & Walberg, H. J. (1987). The effects of computer-based instruction in elementary schools: A quantitative synthesis. *Journal of Research on Computing in Education, 20,* 85–103.

Nowacek, E. J., McKinney, J. D., & Hallahan, D. P. (1990). Instructional behaviors of more or less effective beginning regular and special educators. *Exceptional Children, 57,* 140–149.

Odom, S. L., & Karnes, M. B. (Eds.). (1988). *Early intervention for infants and children with handicaps: An empirical base.* Baltimore: Brookes.

O'Leary, K. D. (1980). Pills or skills for hyperactive children. *Journal of Applied Behavior Analysis, 13,* 191–204.

Osgood, C. E. (1957). Motivational dynamics of language behavior. In M. R. Jones (Ed.), *Nebraska symposium on motivation.* Lincoln: University of Nebraska Press.

Oswald, D. P. (1995). Identification of special education students with mental retardation: Correlates of state child-count data. *Journal of Child and Family Studies, 4,* 389–397.

Patterson, G., DeBaryshe, B. D., & Ramsey, E. (1989). A developmental perspective on antisocial behavior. *American Psychologist, 44,* 329–335.

Patton, J. R., Cronin, M. E., Polloway, E. A., Hutchinson, D., & Robinson, G. (1989). Curricular considerations: A life skills orientation. In G. A. Robinson, J. R. Patton, E. A. Polloway, & L. R. Sargent (Eds.), *Best practices in mild mental disabilities* (pp. 21–38). Reston, VA: Council for Exceptional Children, Division on Mental Retardation.

Patton, J. R., Polloway, E. A., Smith, T. E. C., Edgar, E., Clark, G. M., & Lee, S. (1996). Individuals with mild mental retardation: Postsecondary outcomes and implications for educational policy. *Education and Training in Mental Retardation and Developmental Disabilities, 31,* 75–85.

Pearl, R. (1987). Social cognitive factors in learning-disabled children's social problems. In S. J. Ceci (Ed.), *Handbook of cognitive, social, and neuropsychological aspects of learning disabilities* (pp. 273–294). Hillsdale, NJ: Erlbaum.

Pearl, R. (1992). Psychosocial characteristics of learning disabled students. In N. N. Singh & I. L. Beale (Eds.), *Learning disabilities: Nature, theory, and treatment* (pp. 96–125). San Diego: Academic Press.

Pearpoint, J., & Forest, M. (1992). Foreword. In S. Stainback & W. Stainback (Eds.), *Curriculum considerations in inclusive classrooms: Facilitating learning for all students* (pp. xv–xviii). Baltimore: Brookes.

Pelham, W. E. (1986). The effects of psychostimulant drugs on learning and academic achievement in children with attention-deficit disorders and learning disabilities. In J. Torgesen & B. Wong (Eds.), *Psychological and educational perspectives on learning disabilities* (pp. 160–168). New York: Academic Press.

Perfetti, C. A. (1985). *Reading ability.* New York: Oxford University Press.

Peter, L. J. (1965). *Prescriptive teaching.* New York: McGraw-Hill.

Peterson, P. L., & Walberg, H. J. (Eds.). (1979). *Research on teaching: Concepts, findings, and implications.* Berkeley, CA: McCutchan.

Phillips, D. (1983). After the wake: Post positivistic educational thought. *Educational Researcher, 12,* 4–12.

Phillips, D. C. (1980). What do the researcher and the practitioner have to offer each other? *Educational Researcher, 9,* 17–20, 24.

Polloway, E. A. (1984). The integration of mildly retarded students in the schools: A historical review. *Remedial and Special Education, 5,* 18–28.

Polloway, E. A., Patton, J. R., Smith, J. D., & Roderique, T. W. (1992). Issues in program design for elementary students with mild retardation: Emphasis on curriculum development. *Education and Training in Mental Retardation, 26,* 142–150

Polloway, E. A., & Smith, J. D. (1988). Current status of the mild mental retardation construct: Identification, placement, and programs. In C. Wang, C. Reynolds, & J. Walberg (Eds.), *Handbook of special education: Research and practice* (Vol. 2, pp. 7–22). New York: Pergamon Press.

Polloway, E. A., Smith, J. D., Patton, J. R., & Smith, T. E. C. (1996). Historic changes in mental retardation and developmental disabilities. *Education and Training in Mental Retardation and Developmental Disabilities, 31,* 3–12.

Poplin, M. S. (1988a). Holistic/constructivist principles of the teaching/learning process: Implications for the field of learning disabilities. *Journal of Learning Disabilities, 21,* 389–400.

Poplin, M. S. (1988b). The reductionistic fallacy in learning disabilities: Replicating the past by reducing the present. *Journal of Learning Disabilities, 21,* 401–416.

Pray, B. S., Hall, C. W., & Markley, R. P. (1992). Social skills training: An analysis of social behaviors selected for Individualized Education Programs. *Remedial and Special Education, 13,* 43–49.

Pressley, M., & Harris, K. R. (1990). What we really know about strategy instruction. *Educational Leadership, 48,* 31–34.

Pullis, M. (1985). Temperament characteristics of LD students and their impact on decisions made by resource and mainstream teachers. *Learning Disability Quarterly, 8,* 109–123.

Purkey, S. C., & Smith, M. S. (1983). Effective schools: A review. *Elementary School Journal, 83,* 427–452.

Quay, H. C. (1973). Special education: Assumptions, techniques, and evaluative criteria. *Exceptional Children, 40,* 165–170.

Ramey, C. T., Bryant, D. M., Wasik, B. H., Sparling, J. J., Fendt, K. H., & LaVange, L. M. (1992). The Infant Health and Development Program for low birthweight, premature infants: Program elements, family participation, and child intelligence. *Pediatrics, 89,* 454–465.

Ramey, C. T., & Ramey, S. L. (1992). Effective early intervention. *Mental Retardation, 30,* 337–345.

Reger, R. (1973). What is a resource room program? *Journal of Learning Disabilities, 6,* 607–614.

Reith, H. J., & Evertson, C. (1988). Variables related to the effective instruction of difficult-to-teach children. *Focus on Exceptional Children, 20,* 1–8.

Reynolds, M. C., Wang, M. C., & Walberg, H. J. (1987). The necessary restructuring of special and regular education. *Exceptional Children, 53,* 391–398.

Reynolds, M. C., Wang, M. C., & Walberg, H. J. (1992). The knowledge bases for special and general education. *Remedial and Special Education, 13,* 6–10, 33.

Rimland, B. (1983). The Feingold diet: An assessment of the reviews by Mattes, by Kavale and Forness and others. *Journal of Learning Disabilities, 16,* 331–333.

Rosenberg, M. S., & Jackson, L. (1988). Theoretical models and special education: The impact of varying world views on service delivery and research. *Remedial and Special Education, 9,* 26–34.

Rosenshine, B. (1976). Classroom instruction. In N. L. Gage (Ed.), *The psychology of teaching methods: The seventy-fifth yearbook of the National Society for the Study of Education* (pp. 109–143). Chicago: University of Chicago Press.

Rosenthal, R. (1984). *Meta-analytic procedures for social research.* Beverly Hills, CA: Sage.

Rosenthal, R., & Jacobson, L. (1968). *Pygmalion in the classroom.* New York: Holt, Rinehart & Winston.

Rosenthal, R., & Rubin, D. D. (1978). Interpersonal expectancy effects: The first 345 studies. *Behavioral and Brain Sciences, 3,* 377–415.

Ross, L. E., & Ward, T. B. (1978). The processing of information from short-term visual store: Developmental and intellectual level differences. In N. R. Ellis (Ed.), *International review of research in mental retardation* (Vol. 9, pp. 1–28). New York: Academic Press.

Rutherford, R. B., Chipman, J., DiGangi, S. A., & Anderson, K. (1992). *Teaching social skills: A practical instructional approach.* Ann Arbor, MI: Exceptional Innovations.

Safer, D. J. (1995). Major treatment considerations for attention-deficit hyperactivity disorder. *Current Problems in Pediatrics, 25,* 137–143.

Salomon, G. (1972). Heuristic models for the generation of aptitude-treatment interaction hypotheses. *Review of Educational Research, 42,* 327–343.

Samuels, S. J. (1986). Why children fail to learn and what to do about it. *Exceptional Children, 53,* 7–16.

San Miguel, S. K., Forness, S. R., & Kavale, K. A. (1996). Social skill deficits and learning disabilities: The psychiatric comorbidity hypothesis. *Learning Disability Quarterly, 19,* 252–261.

Schalock, R. L., Stark, J. A., Snell, M. E., Coulter, D. L., Polloway, E. A., Luckasson, R., Reiss, S., & Spitalnik, D. M. (1994). The changing conception of mental retardation: Implications for the field. *Mental Retardation, 32,* 181–193.

Schmidt, M., Weinstein, T., Niemic, R., & Walberg, H. J. (1985–86). Computer-assisted instruction with exceptional children. *Journal of Special Education, 19,* 497–509.

Schneider, B. H., & Byrne, B. M. (1985). Children's social skills training: A meta-analysis. In B. Schneider, K. Rubin, & J. Ledingham (Eds.), *Children's peer relations: Issues in assessment and intervention* (pp. 175–192). New York: Springer-Verlag.

Schrag, P., & Divoky, D. (1975). *The myth of the hyperactive child.* New York: Pantheon.

Schumaker, J. B., & Hazel, J. S. (1988). Social skills and learning disabilities: Current issues and recommendations for future research. In J. Kavanagh & T. Truss (Eds.), *Learning disabilities: Proceedings of the national conference* (pp. 293–344). Parkton, MD: York Press.

Schweinhart, L. J., Berrueta-Clement, J. R., Barnett, W. S., Epstein, A. S., & Weikart, D. P. (1985). Effects of the Perry Preschool Program on youths through age 19: A summary. *Topics in Early Childhood Special Education, 5,* 26–35.

Scruggs, T. E. (1988). Nature of learning disabilities. In K. A. Kavale (Ed.), *Learning disabilities: State of the art and practice* (pp. 22–43). Boston: Little, Brown/College-Hill.

Scruggs, T. E., & Laufenberg, R. (1986). Transformational mnemonic strategies for retarded learners. *Education and Training of the Mentally Retarded, 21,* 165–173.

Scruggs, T. E., & Mastropieri, M. A. (1989). Reconstructive elaborations: A model for content area learning. *American Educational Research Journal, 26,* 311–327.

Scruggs, T. E., & Mastropieri, M. A. (1992). Classroom applications of mnemonic instruction: Acquisition, maintenance, and generalization. *Exceptional Children, 58,* 219–229.

Scruggs, T. E., Mastropieri, M. A., & Levin, J. R. (1985). Vocabulary acquisition of retarded students under direct and mnemonic instruction. *American Journal of Mental Deficiency, 89,* 546–551.

Scruggs, T. E., Mastropieri, M. A., Levin, J. R., & Gaffney, J. S. (1985). Facilitating the acquisition of science facts in learning disabled students. *American Educational Research Journal, 22,* 575–586.

Scruggs, T. E., Mastropieri, M. A., McLoone, B. B., Levin, J. R., & Morrison, C. (1987). Mnemonic facilitation of text-embedded science facts with LD students. *Journal of Educational Psychology, 79,* 27–34.

Scruggs, T. E., & Richter, L. (1985). Tutoring learning disabled students: A critical review. *Learning Disability Quarterly, 8,* 286–298.

Semmel, M. I., Gerber, M. M., & MacMillan, D. S. (1994). Twenty-five years after Dunn's article: A legacy of policy analysis research in special education. *Journal of Special Education, 27,* 481–495.

Shapiro, J. P., Loeb, P., Bowermaster, D., et al. (1993, December 13). Separate and unequal: How special education programs are cheating our children and costing taxpayers billions each year. *U.S. News and World Report, 118,* 46–49, 54–56, 60.

Sheehan, R., & Keogh, B. K. (1984). Approaches to evaluation in special education. In B. K. Keogh (Ed.), *Advances in special education* (Vol. 4, pp. 1–20). Greenwich, CT: JAI Press.

Sheridan, J. J., & Meister, K. A. (1982). *Food additives and hyperactivity.* New York: American Council on Science and Health.

Shonkoff, J. P., & Hauser-Cram, P. (1988). Early intervention for disabled infants and their families. *Pediatrics, 80,* 650–658.

Sindelar, P. T., & Deno, S. L. (1978). The effectiveness of resource programming. *Journal of Special Education, 12,* 17–28.

Skeels, H. M., & Dye, H. B. (1939). A study of the effects of differential stimulation on mentally retarded children. *Proceedings of the American Association on Mental Deficiency, 44,* 114–136.

Skiba, R., & Casey, A. (1985). Interventions for behaviorally disordered students: A quantitative review and methodological critique. *Behavioral Disorders, 10,* 239–252.

Skipper, J. K., Guenther, A. L., & Nass, G. (1967). The sacredness of .05: A note concerning the uses of statistical levels of significance in social science. *American Sociologist, 2,* 16–18.

Slavin, R. (1984). Meta-analysis in education. How has it been used? *Educational Researcher, 13,* 6–15.

Slavin, R. E. (1991). Synthesis of research on cooperative learning. *Educational Leadership, 48,* 71–82.

Slavin, R. E., & Madden, N. A. (1989). What works for students at risk: A research synthesis. *Educational Leadership, 46,* 1–8.

Smart, J. C., & Elton, C. F. (1981). Structural characteristics and citation rates of education journals. *American Educational Research Journal, 18,* 399–414.

Smead, V. S. (1977). Ability training and task analysis in diagnostic-prescriptive teaching. *Journal of Special Education, 11,* 113–125.

Smith, B. C., & West, R. P. (1986). Assessing best practices. *Special Educator, 7,* 6–8.

Smith, J. D. (1994). The revised AAMR definition of mental retardation: The MRDD position. *Education and Training in Mental Retardation and Developmental Disabilities, 27,* 179–183.

Smith, M. L., Glass, G. V., & Miller, T. I. (1980). *The benefits of psychotherapy.* Baltimore: Johns Hopkins University Press.

Smith, T. E. C., & Puccini, I. K. (1995). Position statement: Secondary curriculum policy issues for students with mental retardation. *Education and Training in Mental Retardation and Developmental Disabilities, 30,* 275–282.

Snell, M. E. (1991). Schools are for all kids: The importance of integration for students with severe disabilities and their peers. In J. W. Lloyd, A. C. Repp, & N. N. Singh (Eds.), *The regular education initiative: Alternative perspectives on concepts, issues, and models* (pp. 133–148). Sycamore, IL: Sycamore.

Snider, V. E. (1992a). Learning styles and learning to read: A critique. *Remedial and Special Education, 13,* 6–18.

Snider, V. E. (1992b). Unscientific documentation and philosophical issues: A rejoinder to Carbo. *Remedial and Special Education, 13,* 30–33.

Soltis, J. (1984). On the nature of educational research. *Educational Researcher, 13,* 5–10.

Special ed's special costs. (1993, October 20). *The Wall Street Journal,* p. A14.

Speece, D. L., & Mandell, C. J. (1980). Resource room support services for regular teachers. *Learning Disability Quarterly, 3,* 49–53.

Spitz, H. H. (1963). Field theory in mental deficiency. In N. R. Ellis (Ed.), *Handbook of mental deficiency: Psychological theory and research* (pp. 11–40). New York: McGraw-Hill.

Spitz, H. H. (1966). The role of input organization in the learning and memory of mental retardates. In N. R. Ellis (Ed.), *International review of research in mental retardation* (Vol. 2, pp. 29–57). New York: Academic Press.

Spitz, H. H. (1973a). The channel capacity of educable mental retardates. In D. K. Routh (Ed.), *The experimental psychology of mental retardation* (pp. 133–156). Chicago: Aldine.

Spitz, H. H. (1973b). Consolidating facts into the schematized learning and memory system of educable retardates. In N. R. Ellis (Ed.), *International review of research in mental retardation* (Vol. 6, pp. 149–168). New York: Academic Press.

Spitz, H. H. (1986). *The raising of intelligence: A selected history of attempts to raise retarded intelligence.* Hillsdale, NJ: Erlbaum.

Sprague, R. L., & Werry, J. S. (1971). Methodology of psychopharmacological studies with the retarded. In M. R. Ellis (Ed.), *International review of research in mental retardation: Vol. 5.* New York: Academic Press.

Squires, D. (1983). *Effective schools and classrooms: Research-based perspective.* Alexandria, VA: Association for Supervision and Curriculum Development.

Sroufe, L. A. (1975). Drug treatment of children with behavior problems. In F. J. Horowitz (Ed.), *Review of Child Development Research: Vol. 4.* Chicago: University of Chicago Press.

Stainback, S., & Stainback, W. (1992). *Curriculum considerations in inclusive classrooms: Facilitating learning for all students.* Baltimore: Brookes.

Stare, F. J., Whelan, E. M., & Sheridan, M. (1980). Diet and hyperactivity: Is there a relationship? *Pediatrics, 66,* 521–525.

State, M., King, B. H., & Dykens, E. (1997). Mental retardation: A review of the past 10 years (Part II). *Journal of the American Academy of Child and Adolescent Psychiatry, 36,* 1664–1671.

Sternberg, L., & Taylor, R. L. (1982). The insignificance of psycholinguistic training: A reply to Kavale. *Exceptional Children, 49,* 254–256.

Stevens, R., & Rosenshine, B. (1981). Advances in research on teaching. *Exceptional Education Quarterly, 2,* 1–9.

Stevenson, R. E., Massey, P. S., Schroer, R. J., McDermott, S., & Richter, B. (1996). Preventable fraction of mental retardation: Analysis based on individuals with severe mental retardation. *Mental Retardation, 34,* 182–188.

Strain, P. S., Guralnick, M. J., & Walker, H. M. (1986). *Children's social behavior: Development, assessment, and modification.* New York: Academic Press.

Swanson, H. L. (1984). Does theory guide practice? *Remedial and Special Education, 5*(5), 7–16.

Swanson, H. L., & Malone, S. (1992). Social skills and learning disabilities: A meta-analysis of the literature. *School Psychology Review, 21,* 427–443.

Talbott, E., Lloyd, J. W., & Tankersley, M. (1994). Effects of reading comprehension interventions for students with learning disabilities. *Learning Disability Quarterly, 17,* 223–232.

Talmage, H. (Ed.). (1975). *Systems of individualized education.* Berkeley, CA: McCutchan.

Tarver, S. G., & Dawson, M. M. (1978). Modality preference and the teaching of reading: A review. *Journal of Learning Disabilities, 11,* 5–17.

Taylor, A. M., & Turnure, J. E. (1979). Imagery and verbal elaboration with retarded children: Effects on learning and memory. In N. R. Ellis (Ed.), *Handbook of mental deficiency: Psychological theory and research* (2nd ed., pp. 659–698). Hillsdale, NJ: Erlbaum.

Thormann, M. J., Gersten, R., Moore, L., & Morvant, M. (1986). Microcomputers in special education classrooms: Themes from research and implications for practice. *Computers in the Schools, 3,* 97–109.

Tindal, G. (1985). Investigating the effectiveness of special education: An analysis of methodology. *Journal of Learning Disabilities, 18,* 101–112.

Torgesen, J. K. (1982). The learning disabled child as an inactive learner: Educational implications. *Topics in Learning and Learning Disabilities, 2,* 45–52.

Torgesen, J. K., & Goldman, T. (1977). Rehearsal and short-term memory in reading disabled children. *Child Development, 48,* 389–396.

Torgesen, J. K., & Kail, R. V. (1980). Memory processes in exceptional children. In B. K. Keogh (Ed.), *Advances in special education* (Vol. 1, pp. 55–99). Greenwich, CT: JAI Press.

U.S. Department of Education. (1992). *IDEA Regulations, 34,* C.F.R. 300.552.

Ulman, J. D., & Rosenberg, M. S. (1986). Science and superstition in special education. *Exceptional Children, 52,* 459–460.

Utah Special Education Consortium Evaluation Task Force. (1986). Critical questions for the evaluation of a special education program. *Special Educator, 7,* 3–4.

Van Witsen, B. (1967). *Perceptual training activities handbook.* New York: Teachers College Press.

Vaughn, S. (1991). Social skills enhancement in students with learning disabilities. In B. Y. L. Wong (Ed.), *Learning about learning disabilities* (pp. 407–440). San Diego: Academic Press.

Vaughn, S., & Haager, D. (1994). Social assessments of students with learning disabilities: Do they measure up? In S. Vaughn & C. Bos (Eds.), *Research issues in learning disabilities: Theory, methodology, assessment, and ethics* (pp. 276–311). New York: Springer-Verlag.

Vaughn, S., & Hogan, A. (1994). The social competence of students with learning disabilities over time: A within-individual examination. *Journal of Learning Disabilities, 27,* 292–303.

Vaughn, S., Levine, L., & Ridley, C. (1986). *PALS: Problem-solving and affective learning strategies.* Chicago: Science Research Associates.

Vaughn, S., & Schumm, J. S. (1996). Classroom ecologies: Implications for inclusion of students with learning disabilities. In D. Speece & B. K. Keogh (Eds.), *Research on classroom ecologies: Implications for inclusion of children with learning disabilities.* Hillsdale, NJ: Erlbaum.

Vellutino, F. R., & Scanlon, D. M. (1982). Verbal processing in poor and normal readers. In C. J. Brainerd & M. Pressley (Eds.), *Verbal processes in children: Progress in cognitive development research* (pp. 189–254). New York: Springer-Verlag.

Vockell, E. L., & Mihail, T. (1993). Instructional principles behind computerized instruction for students with exceptionalities. *Teaching Exceptional Children, 25,* 39–43.

Vogel, S., & Forness, S. R. (1992). Social functioning in adults with learning disabilities. *School Psychology Review, 21,* 375–386.

Wachter, K. W., & Straf, M. L. (Eds.). (1990). *The future of meta-analysis.* New York: Russell Sage Foundation.

Wagner, M. (Ed.). (1995). *The national longitudinal transition study of special education students: A summary of findings.* Menlo Park, CA: SRI International.

Walberg, H. J. (1984). Improving the productivity of America's schools. *Educational Leadership, 41,* 19–30.

Walker, H. M., Colvin, G., & Ramsey, E. (1995). *Antisocial behavior in school: Strategies and best practice.* Pacific Grove, CA: Brooks/Cole.

Walker, H. M., & McConnell, S. (1988). *Walker-McConnell scale of social competence and school adjustment.* Austin, TX: PRO-ED.

Walker, H. M., McConnell, S., Holmes, D., Todis, B., Walker, J., & Golden, N. (1983). *The Walker social skills curriculum: The ACCEPTS Program.* Austin, TX: PRO-ED.

Walker, H. M., Street, A., Garrett, B., Crossen, J., Hops, H., & Greenwood, C. R. (1978). *RECESS (Reprogramming environmental contingencies for effective social skills): Manual for consultants.* Unpublished manuscript, Center for Behavioral Education of the Handicapped, University of Oregon, Eugene.

Wang, M. C. (1987). Toward achieving educational excellence for all students: Program design and instructional outcomes. *Remedial and Special Education, 8,* 25–34.

Wang, M. C., & Baker, E. T. (1985–86). Mainstreaming programs: Design features and effects. *Journal of Special Education, 19,* 503–521.

Waxman, H. C., & Walberg, H. J. (1982). The relation of teaching and learning: A review of reviews of process-product research. *Contemporary Education Review, 1,* 103–120.

Waxman, H. C., Wang, M. C., Anderson, K. A., & Walberg, H. J. (1985). Adaptive education and student outcomes: A quantitative synthesis. *Journal of Educational Research, 78,* 228–236.

Weil, M. L., & Murphy, J. (1982). Instructional processes. In H. E. Mitzel (Ed.), *Encyclopedia of educational research* (5th ed., pp. 890–917). New York: Free Press.

Wender, E. H. (1977). Food additives and hyperkinesis. *American Journal of Diseases of Children, 131,* 1204–1206.

Werry, J. S. (1982). An overview of pediatric psychopharmacology. *Journal of the American Academy of Child Psychiatry, 21,* 3–9.

Wesson, C., King, R. P., & Deno, S. L. (1984). Direct and frequent measurement of student performance: If it's good for us, why don't we do it? *Learning Disability Quarterly, 7,* 45–48.

Westling, D. L. (1996). What do parents of children with moderate and severe mental disabilities want? *Education and Training in Mental Retardation and Developmental Disabilities, 31,* 86–114.

White, K. R., Bush, D., & Casto, G. (1986). Let the past be prologue: Learning from previous reviews of early intervention efficacy research. *Journal of Special Education, 19,* 417–428.

White, W. A. T. (1988). A meta-analysis of effects of direct instruction in special education. *Education and Treatment of Children, 11,* 364–374.

Wiederholt, J. L., & Chamberlain, S. P. (1989). A critical analysis of research programs. *Remedial and Special Education, 10,* 15–37.

Wiederholt, J. L., Hammill, D. D., & Brown, V. (1978). *The resource teacher.* Boston: Allyn & Bacon.

Wilens, T. E., & Biederman, J. (1992). The stimulants. *Psychiatric Clinics of North America, 15,* 191–222.

Will, M. (1986). Educating children with learning problems: A shared responsibility. *Exceptional Children, 52,* 411–415.

Wilson, R. (1987). Direct observation of academic learning time. *Teaching Exceptional Children, 19,* 13–17.

Wilson, R., & Wesson, C. (1986). Making every minute count: Academic learning time in LD classrooms. *Learning Disabilities Focus, 2,* 13–19.

Wolf, F. M. (1986). *Meta-analysis: Quantitative methods for research synthesis.* Beverly Hills, CA: Sage.

Ysseldyke, J. E. (1973). Diagnostic-prescriptive teaching: The search for aptitude-treatment interactions. In L. Mann & D. Sabatino (Eds.), *The first review of special education.* Philadelphia: JSE Press.

Ysseldyke, J. E., & Salvia, J. (1974). Diagnostic-prescriptive teaching: Two models. *Exceptional Children, 41,* 181–185.

Ysseldyke, J. E., & Salvia, J. (1980). Methodological considerations in aptitude-treatment interaction research with intact groups. *Diagnostique, 6,* 3–9.

Ysseldyke, J. E., Thurlow, M. L., Christenson, S. L., & Weiss, J. (1987). Time allocated to instruction of mentally retarded, learning disabled, emotionally disturbed, and nonhandicapped elementary students. *Journal of Special Education, 21,* 43–55.

Ysseldyke, J. E., Thurlow, M. L., O'Sullivan, P., & Christenson, S. L. (1989). Teaching structures and tasks in reading instruction for students with mild handicaps. *Learning Disabilities Research, 4,* 78–86.

Zaragoza, N., Vaughn, S., & McIntosh, R. (1991). Social skills interventions and children with behavior problems: A review. *Behavioral Disorders, 16,* 260–275.

Zeaman, D., & House, B. J. (1963). The role of attention in retardate discrimination learning. In N. R. Ellis (Ed.), *Handbook of mental deficiency: Psychological theory and research* (pp. 159–223). New York: McGraw-Hill.

Zeaman, D., & House, B. J. (1979). A review of attention theory. In N. R. Ellis (Ed.), *Handbook of mental deficiency: Psychological theory and research* (2nd ed., pp. 63–120). Hillsdale, NJ: Erlbaum.